# Breaking
# The Cycle

# Breaking The Cycle

## HOW TO TURN CONFLICT INTO COLLABORATION
### When You and Your Patients Disagree

**George F. Blackall, PsyD, MBA**
Associate Professor of Pediatrics and Humanities
The Milton S. Hershey Medical Center
Director of Student Development
Penn State University College of Medicine
Hershey, Pennsylvania

**Steven Simms, PhD**
Associate Director
Philadelphia Child and Family Therapy Training Center
Philadelphia, PA
Independent Practice
Media, PA

**Michael J. Green, MD, MS, FACP**
Professor of Humanities and Medicine
Penn State College of Medicine
Hershey, Pennsylvania

ACP Press®
American College of Physicians • Philadelphia

Associate Publisher and Manager, ACP Press®: Tom Hartman
Production Supervisor: Allan S. Kleinberg
Senior Production Editor: Karen C. Nolan
Publishing Coordinator: Angela Gabella
Cover Design: Lisa Torrieri
Indexer: Kathleen Patterson
Marketing Associate: Caroline Hawkins

Printed in the United States of America
Printing/Binding by McNaughton & Gunn
Composition by Atlis Graphics

**Library of Congress Cataloging-in-Publication Data**

Blackall, George F.
   Breaking the cycle : how to turn conflict into collaboration when you
and your patients disagree / George F. Blackall, Steven Simms, Michael
J. Green.
      p. ; cm.
   Includes bibliographical references and index.
   ISBN 978-1-934465-18-9
 1. Physician and patient.   I. Simms, Steven.   II. Green, Michael J.
(Michael Jay), 1961-   III. American College of Physicians.   IV. Title.
    [DNLM: 1. Physician-Patient Relations.   W 62 B627b 2009]

   R727.3.B52  2009
   610.69'6--dc22

                                                            2009006528
09 10 11 12 13 / 10 9 8 7 6 5 4 3 2 1

# Acknowledgements

One of the themes we stress is that isolation and disconnection from important relationships can lead to psychological distress. Conversely, decreasing isolation and disconnection can lead to productive collaborative relationships. It is the latter that has lead to the completion of this manuscript. While writing a book is a significant challenge, the benefits far outweigh the burdens. In our case, the benefits have come in the form of developing strong collaborative relationships with some extraordinary people.

Tom Hartman, our publisher at the ACP, took a chance on three first-time book authors. His direct, and at times painful, feedback helped shape this manuscript and give it depth. His gift for the English language, and his talent as a teacher, helped us make the leap from academics to book authors. We are extremely grateful.

Lynn Rosen provided the perfect combination of critical assessment, constructive feed-back, strategic advice, and timely inspiration to turn a rough draft into a finished manuscript. Without her, this book would have ended up sitting on a hard drive for eternity. Thank you.

Special thanks to Marla Sussman, who provided keen insights in the developmental editing process. Karen Nolan, our Production Editor, brought a refreshing blend of wisdom, talent, and tact to finish the project.

There have also been many generous colleagues along the way who have given us their time, talent, and wisdom. It is with humility and gratitude that we extend our thanks to: Noel Ballantine, Joe Gesky, John Neely, Cheryl Dellasega, Tom McGarrity, Steve Ross, John Zurlo, John Brendler, Mike Silver, Greg Caputo, Barbara Ostrov, Benjamin Levi, Jen Toth, Karen Bell, and Jeff Gilbert.

Thank you to Barbara Miller, MD, Chief of Pediatric Hematology/Oncology at the Penn State Children's Hospital, and the Four Diamonds Fund, for providing ongoing support and resources that have made this manuscript possible. Richard Simons, MD, Vice Chair for Medical Education at the Penn State University College of Medicine, has generously supported the idea for this project since its inception.

Special thanks to Anne E. Kazak, Ph.D., at the Children's Hospital of Philadelphia, for introducing Drs. Simms and Blackall, and for creating a supportive environment that fostered systems thinking. Additional thanks to the members of the Division of Oncology for providing the context for the development of the ideas that resulted in this manuscript.

Others who provided thoughtful feedback on early versions of the manuscript include Eileen Blackall, Lisa Plotkin, Karen Kline, and Jim Ryan. Thank you for your insights.

Finally, thank you to the most giving teachers we will ever have: our patients.

# Dedication

*To Harry and Patrick, my heroes. Thank you for teaching me about love. And to my dear wife Colleen, thank you for saying "Yes."*    GFB

*To Marion Lindblad-Goldberg and Wayne Jones for giving me the opportunity to sharpen my thinking, to Joe Micucci for helping me to truly understand systems thinking, to John Brendler for nurturing me to become the therapist and teacher that I am today, and, most importantly, to my wife Christine, who instills heart felt meaning in our life.*    SS

*To Lisa, who provided inspiration, encouragement, and insight into this project from its inception, and to my colleagues and patients who have always been my teachers.*    MJG

# Introduction

In 1998, a shy, athletic, twelve-year-old girl with long brown hair and wire-rimmed glasses was diagnosed with acute lymphoblastic leukemia. Her subsequent struggle to swallow life-saving medication set in motion a series of events that resulted in this book. Bridget's inability to take her medicine mobilized a small army of caregivers, all with the same primary goal. Her parents, nurses, doctors, a psychologist, and even the woman who cleaned her hospital room, all tried to coax, reward, threaten, and even beg her to take the drugs. Everyone had a theory that was sure to work. They were all wrong.

What was clear during that several-week struggle was that, while everyone agreed on the desired outcome, no one agreed on how to get there. When the traditional methods failed—methods such as crushing the pills into chocolate pudding, or rewarding her for taking the pills—there was no Plan B. As Bridget continued unsuccessfully to try to take her medicines, her parents and caregivers were rendered utterly helpless.

The failed attempts to help Bridget are one example of the sort of impasse that can develop between doctors and patients. Doctors want to help their patients, and they utilize all of their knowledge, skills, and experience to this end. Patients, in turn, want to be helped by their doctors. They seek out medical expertise for the purpose of diagnosing and hopefully resolving medical problems. In most cases, the system of patients seeking aid and advice from doctors and doctors providing this assistance works smoothly. Where possible, medical issues are resolved in a satisfactory manner. Sometimes, however, as with the case of Bridget, things do not flow so smoothly. Despite the best efforts of both patient and doctor, sometimes bumps occur in the process that can make it hard to navigate, or even hard to understand. After all, why would an ill young girl struggle so mightily to take her medication? And yet struggle she did.

Sometimes the impasses doctors face are about small issues; other times they relate to problems that are truly about life and death. And often, when doctors come to these impasses, they get stuck, as did Bridget's caretakers. After using all of their resources to no effect, they didn't know where to turn next. In Bridget's case, her psychologist, Dr. George Blackall, realized that he was outmatched by a twelve-year-old. Desperate, he called a friend and colleague, Dr. Steve Simms, for help. Steve, a psychologist who had been studying systems interventions for families in trouble with master family therapist John Brendler, suggested a framework to understand, approach, and ultimately resolve the impasse between Bridget and her caregivers. It is the framework that he suggested that has led to this book.

The framework Steve recommended is called the "Symptomatic Cycle," and in the ten years since that hot, frustrating summer, George and Steve have worked together to expand this approach used in family therapy for use in doctor/patient relationships. This work led to the development of the Physician-as-Collaborator Model, which we rely on to resolve impasses between doctors and patients. In 2000, Dr. Michael Green joined us, adding his perspective as a practicing internist and medical ethicist. Since then, we have successfully used the Symptomatic Cycle framework and the Physician-as-Collaborator Model thousands of times to help understand and resolve a wide variety of problems in doctor/patient relationships. This approach has become our Plan A, essentially eliminating the need for a Plan B.

In this book, we will demonstrate how to successfully use the Physician-as-Collaborator Model to resolve doctor/patient impasses. We will begin by illustrating the underlying structure of the doctor/patient relationship. By showing how this relationship works, we hope to demonstrate how impasses arise and then how to navigate and resolve them. On the pages ahead you will meet doctors and patients who are stuck in a variety of impasses. You will see how the physicians struggle with their patients and, ultimately, how they use our models to overcome their frustrations and resolve their impasses.

While the sources of frustration faced by physicians in daily practice are numerous (insurance companies, paperwork, malpractice worries, regulations, etc.), our focus is on the relationships with patients that have reached an impasse. Our aim is to help doctors successfully navigate difficult patient encounters that can evolve into cycles of conflict and struggles for control. By using a therapeutic process based on "systems principles" from family therapy, we will present models that focus on three main areas: 1) seeing/recognizing, 2) understanding, and 3) responding to difficult relationships in clinical medicine. This is *not* a book that will tell you how to "get the patient to change." In fact, we will do just the opposite. The focus will be on how changes in the *physician's* thinking can help improve challenging interactions with patients and their families.

For example, imagine receiving a telephone call one busy afternoon from Deborah Rowland. Her husband Al is a long-standing patient of yours and he has a drinking problem. Deborah has called numerous times in the past, and as with prior calls, today she pleads with you to "do something" to help her husband stop drinking. As the conversation progresses, Deborah becomes increasingly agitated and angry. As a physician, you can interpret her anger in several ways. One way is to view Deborah's behavior as rude and disrespectful. If that view dominates your thinking, the natural response will be to become tense and try to control or pull away from her. An alternative way to view her behavior is as the frightened and desperate response of a woman who feels powerless to help her husband. If you have this understanding, you will be more likely to respond in an open and nurturing manner. While Deborah's behavior is the same in both scenarios, your response to her behavior is quite different.

Even when physicians try hard to respond to patients in thoughtful ways, impasses with patients and families inevitably occur. We bring the collective experience of an internist, a health psychologist, and a family therapist to help resolve these impasses. In our combined experiences working at a variety of academic medical centers, we have been impressed by the interpersonal skills that physicians harness to help their patients and their families. Despite witnessing the stresses of pain, suffering, and even death, the vast majority of physicians are humane and compassionate with their patients. They are smart, motivated, and caring people who do their best to help. Yet, even when physicians have motivation and compassion, problems still occur. There are times when these situations escalate, and ruptures develop in relationships. As emotions flare, physicians feel isolated and ineffective, leaving them wondering: "How did these problems develop? What can I do to prevent them?" We will present two models that will help answer those questions.

The first model is the traditional model of the doctor-patient relationship. We call it the "Physician-as-Expert Model," and it is described in detail in Chapter 1. In this model, the doctor listens, diagnoses, and prescribes with the intent of helping the patient feel better. The patient, hoping to feel better, follows the doctor's recommendation. This model generally works well and is the most common way that doctors interact with patients. But sometimes the Physician-as-Expert Model gets derailed by a stalemate that develops between the patient and the physician. When these impasses persist, they lead to repeating patterns of frustration and counterproductive behaviors.

In Chapter 2 we introduce the "Symptomatic Cycle" as a framework to help physicians see and overcome the forces that perpetuate frustrating impasses. We use this framework as a map to guide physicians as they develop strategies for resolving difficult encounters in their daily practice. This framework also serves as the bridge between the Physician-as-Expert Model and our second model, The Physician-as-Collaborator.

In Chapter 3 we describe the Physician-as-Collaborator Model, which views the patient and physician as partners in the process of trying to achieve the patient's health goals. Each partner brings expertise to the relationship, and this Model demonstrates how to best use that expertise to help the patient. This is where we help a physician determine a course of action by describing specific principles that can be applied with patients and their families.

In Chapter 4, we present some basic guidelines for effectively communicating with patients and their families that, if used, will improve your clinical skills and help to prevent many impasses. Yet even when a physician has strong communication skills, impasses can still occur.

In Chapters 5 through 10 we apply the models and principles to difficult cases to bring it all together in a way that busy practitioners can use in daily practice. For example, in Chapters 5 and 6 we introduce two patients who are each driving their physicians to their wits end. Both patients have chronic medical problems, and their physicians are frustrated by the increasing demands being placed upon them. Chapter 7 addresses the problem of chronic pain in a pediatric patient, while Chapter 8 illustrates how to use our models in a crisis in the intensive care unit. Chapter 9 deals with a thorny ethical issue around a patient's wish to die, and Chapter 10 demonstrates how to successfully apply the models to a patient with multiple medical complaints driven by considerable psychological factors.

All of these cases have practical and generalizable aspects that can be applied to a range of different cases, not just the ones presented in the chapters. When we teach medical students how to handle difficult encounters with patients and families, they often say: "Teaching us about communication is nice. Learning about theories of human behavior is fine, too. But what we really need to know is, how do we use these theories in our daily work with patients?" The way we help medical students is the same way we will help you. We use clinical case examples to illustrate how impasses develop and how our models can be used to understand and resolve the gridlock. The cases are drawn from our experiences and combine actual with fictitious patient encounters. Some cases have been adapted from interviews with physician colleagues who generously shared their experiences with us. Others are our own, with personal details altered to protect the privacy of patients and caregivers. Our goal is to provide physicians with a clear, practical, and engaging book that will offer a new understanding and set of skills to respond to and help patients.

Whether the challenge arises in a routine office visit or the ICU, whether it is pediatrics or geriatrics, the tools we present in this book will enable physicians to overcome challenges and bring greater insight and skills to their practice of medicine.

# Contents

# Part I
# Seeing the Cycle

# Chapter 1

# Doctor Knows Best (Sometimes): The "Physician-as-Expert" Model

Annette Sansom knew she wanted to be a physician from the time she was eight years old. As a child, she would pretend to perform an operation to save a neighborhood child's life, or mix a special medicine to help her friend's father with a cough.

Once in medical school, Annette decided on a career in internal medicine because the variety of medical problems that internists see offered the opportunity to develop long-term relationships with patients. Though not a star in medical school, she always excelled in dealing with patients. Her clerkship evaluations were filled with comments like "quickly develops rapport with patients," "sought out by patients," and "able to deal with even the most difficult of patients."

---

**Key Terms**

- Physicians are Human
- Thoughts Drive Behavior
- Physician-as-Expert
- Impasses in the Doctor-Patient Relationship

---

Yet despite Dr. Sansom's obvious "people skills," there were still times, even after five years of practice, that she would end up in a disagreement with a patient and not know how it happened, or even worse, what to do to resolve it. One of her patients, Rich Wilson, is a good example.

Rich Wilson is a 43-year-old former carpenter with a history of multiple back surgeries, each of which worsened his chronic back pain. He is considered to have Failed Back Syndrome, is on disability, and takes daily narcotics to manage his pain. He visits the clinic monthly and is demanding and, at times, antagonistic toward the medical staff. Some of the office staff wonder whether he is milking the system. When Dr. Sansom sees his name on the schedule, she mutters under her breath: "This is going to take forever."

Dr. Sansom feels guilty for having such a visceral and negative reaction to seeing Mr. Wilson's name on her schedule. She remembers an esteemed professor in medical school, in his starched white coat, pronouncing the need for "clinical detachment" in all patient encounters. Somehow she had never been able to master being detached from her patients. In talking about Mr. Wilson to a trusted colleague, she attempts to analyze her reaction. "He just gets under my skin. I try hard not to feel so negative, but I do. I feel guilty about it, but after a while I get mad. I think, what right does he have to bully the nurses and give me such an attitude? He acts like we owe him something. It's not like we aren't trying to help him. He's looking for some magical fix, but some things in medicine simply aren't fixable." While judging herself harshly for having negative feelings toward her patient, what Dr. Sansom does not realize is that she is not alone in her predicament.

# The Physician as a Human Being

All physicians have both good and bad feelings about their patients. Since feelings are a normal part of patient encounters, the goal of remaining "detached" is misguided. Although we like to think that our personal feelings (both positive and negative) do not influence patient care, a handful of studies suggest otherwise (1-4). When physicians like their patients, there is a higher likelihood that their patients will report being satisfied with the physicians (5). Both doctors and patients can tell, better than chance, whether the other person liked them (5). Further studies show that doctors like healthy patients more than sick ones (6,7), and feelings of frustration and anger in response to angry or demanding patients are common (8).

What these studies tell us is that physicians are human beings and as such, they exist in a social context that is broader than the doctor-patient relationship. That context contains conflicting roles and responsibilities that can result in the physician feeling frustrated, which in turn can end up being expressed toward the patient. Physicians also experience multiple forces that shape their feelings and behavior. For example, in addition to Dr. Sansom's patient-care responsibilities, she has obligations to her husband and two children. Some physicians have obligations to students and research. All doctors must consider how laws and economic forces influence practice. It is important to recognize that such competing obligations are common and inevitable. It is how a physician thinks about these conflicts that is an important factor in determining the outcome.

## Thoughts Drive Behavior

Difficult cases like Dr. Sansom's may not have medical answers and seem to lack any interpersonal solutions. They are characterized by patterns of frustration and emotional escalation or withdrawal. The way a physician *thinks* about such cases shapes the way he or she understands and responds to them (9). Consider what happens when Dr. Sansom has the office visit she was dreading with Mr. Wilson. In their interaction, you will see how the negative feelings experienced and expressed by each of them contribute toward moving the relationship to an impasse.

## "This Pain Is Killing Me!"

Mr. Wilson is a person who tries the patience of even the most humane physicians. Although Dr. Sansom believes that Mr. Wilson is in pain, she also suspects that he could do a lot more to help himself.

For today's visit, Dr. Sansom enters the exam room with a knot in her stomach. Nevertheless, she greets Mr. Wilson with a warm smile and extends her hand. He shakes her hand dismissively and eagerly responds to her first question asking how he is today.

> *"Terrible! This pain is killing me. I take the medicines, but nothing helps. I don't know how much longer I can take this. Those criminals at the worker's comp board are trying to take away my benefits. I don't know how they think a man's supposed to live."*

Dr. Sansom recoils at the intensity of his complaints. She remains calm, however, and tries to stay in her role as an expert by assessing whether his pain had changed since the last visit.

> *"It's worse! I can tell doctor, its getting worse. I can't sleep, my wife says I'm miserable to live with (she's no picnic, either, by the way) and all I do is lay around the house all day. You've got to help me, doc."*

Mr. Wilson's request for help appeals to Dr. Sansom's expertise. The problem is that her medical expertise can only take them so far. Dr. Sansom feels a sense of powerlessness and even wonders if she is failing Mr. Wilson. The paradox of feeling a sense of failure is that, as the expert, Sansom feels compelled to do more, yet deep down knows that her allopathic bag of tricks is, essentially, empty.

How a physician responds to feelings of powerlessness and failure is a key to determining the outcome. The need to "do something" (prescribe another medicine, order more tests) may temporarily soothe the anxiety in the relationship with the patient, but ultimately it may further the frustrating cycle. In some cases, the situation will improve. Prescribing a higher dose of narcotics for a patient complaining of persistent pain may well bring relief. But other times, despite the physician's genuine efforts, no progress is made. Both parties then feel "stuck" and despite the best efforts of the patient and physician, there is no movement.

When relationships get stuck, one response is to withdraw (10), which can lead to deterioration in the relationship. The patient's reaction to the withdrawal then exacerbates the situation; when patients sense that the physician is withdrawing, they may become frightened and feel betrayed, which leads to further deterioration in the relationship. It is this deterioration that contributes to the withdrawal and resultant impasse.

Dr. Sansom feels stuck with Mr. Wilson, yet also feels responsible as "the expert" and continues to try to offer something to help him. She thinks for a moment, then suggests returning to physical therapy.

Mr. Wilson has strong beliefs about that suggestion. "No way, Dr. Sansom. Those people are medieval torturers. I won't go back there again. What else can you do?" Feeling frustrated, Dr. Sansom then suggests that Mr. Wilson go to a local pain clinic. Mr. Wilson feels the sting of rejection and asks Dr. Sansom if she is dumping him. She replies somewhat defensively: "I am just trying to find some help for you."

Dr. Sansom feels more guilt because Mr. Wilson sensed that she wanted to get rid of him. As she thought about it, she realized that she didn't want to get rid of him as much as she wanted to feel like she was doing something to help him. Because she felt powerless, she started to withdraw emotionally from Mr. Wilson. It was her emotional withdrawal that kept her locked in the unsatisfying cycle with Mr. Wilson. The more she withdrew, the more he demanded.

## Physician-as-Expert

The field of cognitive psychology shows how thoughts drive feelings, as in the situation described above. These feelings in turn, ultimately shape our behavior (11). Dr. Sansom's negative thoughts about Mr. Wilson ("He's milking the system"; "He's going to take forever"; "I can't help this guy") generate negative feelings, which then influence how she interacts with him. She struggles with Mr. Wilson because he frustrates her by challenging the typical way she practices medicine. She is not accustomed to experiencing resistance from patients, especially the type she experiences from Mr. Wilson. Sansom is used to assuming the role of expert and using her knowledge and skills to guide her patients back to health. This pattern of interaction is what we call the Physician-as-Expert Model. It is presented as the starting point for understanding how relationships get stuck, leaving the physician in a bind of not knowing how to help her patient or herself (Figure 1-1).

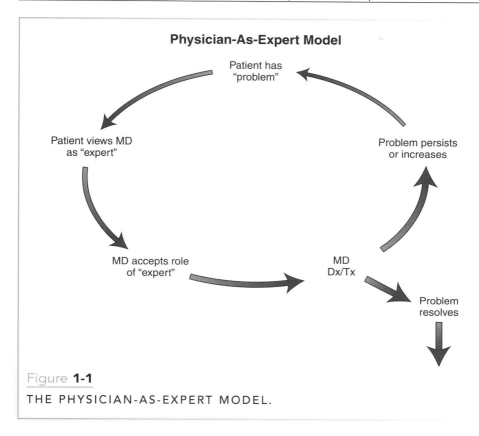

**Figure 1-1**

THE PHYSICIAN-AS-EXPERT MODEL.

In this traditional model of the doctor-patient relationship, the patient seeks out the physician because she possesses the knowledge and skills to help the patient feel better. When this model works—and it usually works quite well—it can be gratifying for both the patient and the physician. The patient gets what he wants and the physician feels like she has helped her patient. This model is enacted countless times each day in clinics and hospitals throughout the world. In some cases however, the model breaks down.

# Model Breakdown: How the Physician-as-Expert Model Fails

The Physician-as-Expert Model breaks down if a doctor and patient persistently disagree on either the underlying cause of the presenting symptom and/or on the best way to proceed. In and of itself, disagreements between doctors and patients are not necessarily a problem and, in fact, are quite common (12). Conflicts occur in all aspects of interpersonal relationships, and most people have a reasonable set of skills to resolve the issues. For example, a physician may want a patient to return for a follow-up visit in one week.

The patient may feel like a one-week return visit is unnecessary and a waste of time and money. The two parties then discuss their different views and ultimately reach an agreement they both can live with. The relationship is unharmed by the conflict and they are able to continue to work together.

In some cases, conflict can even be good for the doctor-patient relationship. We recently had a case where a 23-year-old woman with non-Hodgkins lymphoma arrived in tears at the outpatient clinic for chemotherapy. She told her nurse: "I can't do this today. I don't have the energy for it. I want to feel good for the weekend when I see my boyfriend and the chemo will ruin that for me." When the physician heard about this he became irritated and defensive telling her that, "You need this chemotherapy today." After seeing a few other patients and talking to some colleagues, the physician began to reconsider his position. He went in to see the patient and asked her to tell him more about why she was refusing chemotherapy. After a long discussion he felt like she was making a reasonable decision and agreed with her, even though he was concerned that she would refuse treatment the following week. Since that time, the doctor and patient have been able to talk more openly and freely.

Unlike the above case, an impasse develops when the disagreement *persists* and the relationship between the doctor and the patient begins to *deteriorate*. This is when the Physician-as-Expert Model breaks down. In the case of Mr. Wilson, the patient with Failed Back Syndrome, Dr. Sansom's relationship with him is heading toward an impasse as he persists in making demands on her that she feels unable to meet.

# Impasses in the Doctor-Patient Relationship

What happens to the Physician-as-Expert Model when an impasse is reached, like the one between Mr. Wilson and Dr Sansom? When a physician tries hard to help the patient but sees that his or her efforts are not working, she can become quite frustrated. When this happens, the physician is faced with feeling *responsible*—after all, the physician is the expert—but *powerless* to fulfill that responsibility. Often it is the physician's feeling of powerlessness that leads to emotional withdrawal, which can then fuel an impasse. Figure 1-2 illustrates this concept.

Dr. Sansom was feeling powerless in her interactions with Mr. Wilson. This case illustrates how easy it is to become caught in a cycle of frustration and a resultant impasse with a patient. While she approached each visit with the best of intentions, somehow they always ended with her feeling guilty and powerless and with Mr. Wilson asking for more than she could provide.

Dr. Sansom's interactions with Mr. Wilson have helped us understand what happens when a physician sticks to a model that no longer works. In the remaining chapters, stories of other doctors and patients will help us further understand how impasses develop and what can be done to resolve them. In Chapter 2, we will introduce the Symptomatic Cycle, which will provide a framework that explains how impasses are created and sustained.

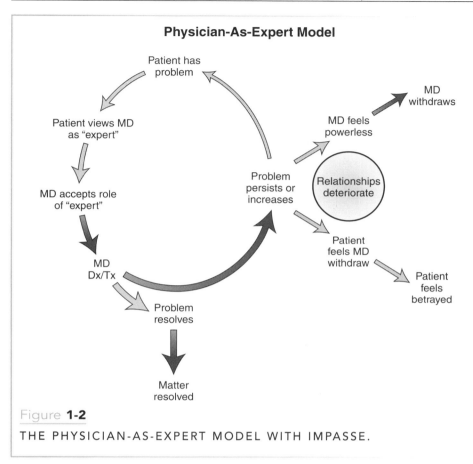

**Physician-As-Expert Model**

Figure **1-2**

THE PHYSICIAN-AS-EXPERT MODEL WITH IMPASSE.

The psychotherapist Jay Haley once purportedly wrote; "The solution of an impasse turns upon a paradox: to confess failure is to begin to move; to experience impotence is to be set free to take action" (13).

**Summary**

In this chapter we have presented:

- The model of Physician-as-Expert
- How unproductive impasses between doctors and patients can evolve
- How the unproductive cycle can lead to deterioration in the relationship, which in turn can produce an impasse

# References

1. **Zinn WM.** Doctors have feelings too. JAMA. 1988;259:3296-8.

2. **Gorlin R, Zucker HD.** Physicians' reactions to patients: a key to teaching humanistic medicine. N Engl J Med. 1983;308:1059-63.

3. **Levinson W.** Mining for gold. J Gen Intern Med. 1993;8:172.

4. **Krebs EE, Konrad TR.** The difficult doctor? Characteristics of physicians who report frustration with patients: an analysis of survey data. BMC Health Serv Res. 2006;6:128.

5. **Levinson W, Frankel RM, Roter DL, Drum M.** How much do surgeons like their patients? Patient Education Counseling. 2006;61:429-34.

6. **Hall J, Horgan TG, Stein TS, Roter DL.** Liking in the physician-patient relationship. Patient Education Counseling. 2002;48:69-77.

7. **Hall JA, Epstein AM, DeCiantis ML, McNeil BJ.** Physicians' liking for their patients: more evidence for the role of affect in medical care. Health Psychol. 1993;12:140-6.

8. **Levinson W, Stiles WB, Inui TS, Engle R.** Physician frustration in communicating with patients. Med Care. 1993;31:285-95.

9. **Groopman J.** How Doctors Think. New York: Houghton Mifflin; 2007.

10. **Neill JR, Kniskern DP, eds.** From Psyche to System: The Evolving Therapy of Carl Whitaker. New York: The Guilford Press; 1982.

11. **Beck AT.** Cognitive therapy: a 30-year retrospective. Am Psychologist. 1991;46:368-75.

12. **Studdert DM, Burns JP, Mello MM, et al.** Nature of conflict in the care of pediatric intensive care patients with prolonged stay. Pediatrics. 2003;112:553-8.

13. **Neill JR, Kniskern DP, eds.** From Psyche to System: The Evolving Therapy of Carl Whitaker. New York: The Guilford Press; 1982:38.

# Part II
# Understanding Unproductive Cycles in Relationships

# Chapter 2
# The Harder I Try, The Worse It Gets: The Symptomatic Cycle

Renowned family therapist Salavador Minuchin writes in *Families and Family Therapy* about "an informal seminar that was held twice a day for thirty to forty minutes over more than two years as Jay Haley, Bruno Mantalvo, and I were driving to and from the Philadelphia Child Guidance Clinic" (1). That "informal seminar" further developed and crystallized into a school of thought and practice called Structural Family Therapy, which revolutionized the way psychotherapists attempt to understand and help families in distress. His writings continue to influence practice today (2). Minuchin's basic tenet was that focusing solely on the individual who was in distress was too limiting because it excluded the rich source of data and support that was available from the primary social context for that person: mainly, the family. He argued quite convincingly that influencing the context within

**Key Terms**
- Symptom
- Symptomatic Cycle

which a person existed could have a powerful effect on an individual's feelings and behavior. He went on to successfully apply this model to a variety of medical and mental health issues, including patients with diabetes and with anorexia (3).

Minuchin observed that focusing exclusively on getting an anorectic child to eat was problematic because it missed the influence of important family dynamics on the child's decision to avoid food. He describes one family, the Gilberts, whose parents were petrified that their 15-year-old daughter with anorexia was going to die (3). The Gilberts portray their family as normal until their daughter was changed by the illness. Minuchin described one therapy session:

"The therapist meets with the family at lunch and they all eat together. The therapist asks the parents to help their daughter survive by making her eat. The daughter refuses to eat and responds to her parents with a broad range of surprisingly sophisticated insults. The therapist focuses on these insults, pointing out that the daughter is strong enough to defeat both parents. The parents close ranks. The parents and therapist together demand that the daughter, who is suddenly perceived as strong, competent, and stubborn, monitor her own body" (4).

By using the power of relationships, Minuchin shows how this realignment can evoke change.

Dr. Steve Simms learned early in his career about the power of using relationships to help people change and re-establish important connections in life. Steve describes an important early career experience:

> *"I had just finished my internship training and had started a course of advanced study in family therapy at the Philadelphia Child Guidance Clinic. I was studying under a number of structural family therapists, including my mentor, John Brendler, a student of Minuchin. I was required to be on call for psychiatric emergencies that were brought to the Children's Hospital of Philadelphia (CHOP), next door. One late October afternoon I was feeling relieved and a bit lucky because I had 15 minutes remaining on my shift, and I hadn't had to deal with any psychiatric emergencies that day. Then my beeper went off, and I knew my luck had run out.*
>
> *"Takita was a 10-year-old girl who was taken by ambulance to CHOP after suddenly losing her ability to walk after she fell at school earlier in the day. She had an extensive neurological work-up, and the attending physician believed that Takita had a conversion disorder. I met her mother and aunt in the emergency department. Takita's history was unremarkable, except that about a month before this incident several cousins began to live in her home. I thought that this was relevant to the onset of her symptoms, but I wasn't sure. I felt*

*as if I needed a few minutes to think through how best to respond to Takita and her mother, so I excused myself and went to the library at the Philadelphia Child Guidance Clinic to do some research.*

*"When I got to the library, most of the staff had gone home for the day, so I was on my own. As I opened a psychiatry textbook, I was struck by one sentence that suggested that traditional medical approaches to helping patients with conversion disorders—extensive medical testing and work-up—might inadvertently and unintentionally reinforce the conversion symptoms. That sentence inspired me to trust what I had recently been taught about the basic principles of structural family therapy [which will be presented in Chapter 3].*

*"My working hypothesis was that the disruption of having cousins join her household had impinged on Takita's relationship with her mother. Instead of focusing exclusively on Takita (i.e., "She must be depressed; put her on meds" or "She's faking the paralysis; set up a behavior modification program with strong enough positive reinforcements and she will walk"), I focused on trying to help Takita and her mother to reconnect. Despite pressure from the medical staff for a psychiatric admission, I told Takita's mother to take her home, warm some milk on the stove, and let Takita sit on her lap as she drank the warm milk. I set up an appointment to see them the next morning. Our agreement was that if there were no improvement in Takita's condition, she would be admitted to the psychiatric hospital.*

*"Takita's mother called me at 8 a.m. the following morning and told me: 'She's walking. I don't need to bring her in.' She thought it was a miracle. I thought it was time to find more ways to use this approach and framework in medical settings."*

# The Symptomatic Cycle

"Symptom" is one of the most familiar words in a physician's vocabulary. For our purposes, "symptom" is used to refer to a wide range of problems (behavioral and medical) that lock the patient/family/physician system in an unproductive struggle that leads to an impasse. A symptom can include a patient being chronically late for appointments or the demand for narcotics to treat questionable pain complaints. The net effect of the problematic behavior is that it entangles the patient/family/physician system around an unremitting medical problem and/or behavior that is troubling to the physician.

Symptoms are connected to systems (5,6). For example, severe pain can impact the cardiovascular system by increasing heart rate and blood pressure.

Likewise, shortness of breath can impact the central nervous system and cause anxiety and light headedness. The relationship between symptoms and systems is well established in human physiology. That same relationship has not been so obvious in the context of human behavior.

Work by Minuchin (1,3) and other writings by Lynn Hoffman (7) introduced the idea that there is often a functional relationship between an identified behavioral symptom (anorexia, non-adherence in diabetes, aggressive behavior) and the family system. This work showed and reinforced the notion that focusing on the individual as an isolated entity excluded the power of the family system in shaping behavior. Early family therapists, including John Brendler and Michael Silver, recognized patterns of behavior in troubled relationships and explained it using a model they called the "Symptomatic Cycle" (6). This work was further clarified, and strategies for disrupting unproductive cycles of behavior were articulated in *The Adolescent in Family Therapy: Breaking the Cycle of Conflict and Control* by Joseph Micucci (8), a psychologist and supervisor of Steve Simms at the Philadelphia Child Guidance Clinic.

Others, including Susan McDaniel (9) and John Rolland (10), started to apply family systems models to patients who suffered from medical illnesses. Anne Kazak at The Children's Hospital of Philadelphia, a mentor to both Steve and George, did groundbreaking work in the application of family systems models to children with cancer and their families (11-14). Steve, George, and eventually Michael Green, extended this work to another context and began using it directly with physicians and nurses to help them become more effective in dealing with difficult patient encounters (15-16).

## Symptoms Drive the Cycle

The Physician-as-Expert Model showed how disagreements or conflict can lead to emotional withdrawal, which can then potentially lead to an impasse. The breakdown of the Physician-as-Expert Model marks the onset of the Symptomatic Cycle. The Symptomatic Cycle framework shows how impasses are *sustained*. One can think of the Symptomatic Cycle as a map that puts a troubling "symptom" in the context of important relationships. Like an actual map, the Symptomatic Cycle provides a broad overview of a landscape, but to successfully use it, one must get feedback from the environment (road signs, directional markers) and make adjustments accordingly. The map of the Symptomatic Cycle is intended to guide physicians through the difficult terrain of conflicted relationships with patients.

As the physician feels increasingly powerless in the face of an impasse, he or she pulls away from the relationship with his or her patient. The relationship between the doctor and the patient then deteriorates as each party focuses on the presenting symptom. Thus the *symptom* distracts people from the *relationship* (the system).

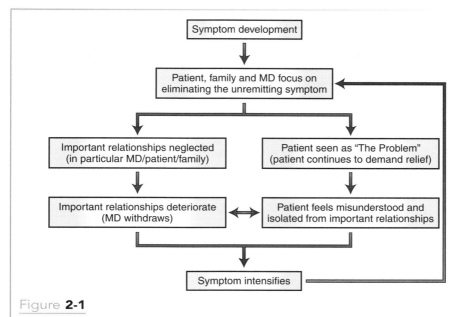

Figure **2-1**

**THE SYMPTOMATIC CYCLE.**
From Micucci JA. The Adolescent in Family Therapy: Breaking the Cycle of Conflict and Control. New York: The Guilford Press; 1998:18; with permission.

Our purposes in using the Symptomatic Cycle here are to create a visual image of interpersonal conflicts and to de-emphasize distracting symptoms in favor of relationships. Our goal is to help you use this model to focus less on the "problem" and more on the relationship with the patient. This change in focus will help you to transition from over-reliance on the Physician-as-Expert Model and build confidence for using the Physician-as-Collaborator Model, which will be presented in Chapter 3. A schematic view of the Symptomatic Cycle is presented in Figure 2-1.

The Symptomatic Cycle framework illustrates how focusing on the "symptom" reduces attention to important relationships, which paradoxically, escalates the symptom. Whatever the symptom, the physician is faced with the dilemma of trying hard to help the patient, yet feeling increasingly frustrated, powerless, and ineffective because the patient continues to complain that problems have not been solved. The following example will help to illustrate the usefulness of the model in clinical practice.

## Applying the Symptomatic Cycle

Robert Hanson has been practicing medicine for 10 years. He is a high-energy person who enjoys seeing patients and likes to move through the day at a steady pace. On good days, he finishes up at an hour that lets him get to the driving range, if not actually play a few holes on his favorite local golf course.

Today he is seeing one of his newer patients, Charlie Reed. Mr. Reed has a cold and is insisting on receiving antibiotics.

> **Mr. Reed begins,** *"Oh, Dr. Hanson, I've got this terrible sore throat, my nose won't stop running, and my head is pounding like a bass drum."*

> **Dr. Hanson conducts a thorough exam and says as empathetically as possible,** *"You must be pretty uncomfortable, Mr. Reed, but it seems as if you have a common cold. The best thing for you now is to get rest and drink plenty of fluids. You should be feeling better in a few days. Feel free to take aspirin or over-the-counter medicines like Tylenol Cold and Flu or Nyquil. They should help you get a bit more comfortable and also help you sleep."*

> **Mr. Reed presses his case,** *"I've tried those things, but they don't work very well. Dr. Hanson, I understand what you are saying, but I feel really bad. In the past, I've been put on an antibiotic, amoxa-something I think, and it really helped. I'm down for the count right now, and I think it's bad enough to get some medicine."*

> **Dr. Hanson responds,** *"Well, common colds tend to run their course in 7 to 10 day, and antibiotics really don't help cure colds. I think your best chance for getting some relief is to try the over-the-counter medicines that I mentioned. Prescribing antibiotics for this will have little effect. Also, there are potential long-term consequences of being repeatedly on antibiotics."*

> **Mr. Reed persists,** *"Oh, sure, I've read about those bugs that are so strong that no medicine can kill them. But I've also read a lot about people who don't get antibiotics when they need them and they get into real trouble, too. Why won't you help me with this one?"*

Dr. Hanson, the expert, knows that antibiotics will not cure Mr. Reed's cold. Yet Mr. Reed is convinced that antibiotics will help him feel better. To frame this dilemma using the Symptomatic Cycle, the "symptom" is Mr. Reed's demand for antibiotics (Figure 2-2).

Focusing on the symptom (the request for antibiotics), Dr. Hanson feels compelled to explain to Mr. Reed *why* antibiotics will not help cure a cold. This is exactly what he is supposed to do when acting in the role of expert, and in many cases this is adequate. The patient accepts the explanation and the matter is resolved. However, sometimes, like in Mr. Reed's case, this explanation does not satisfy the patient. In fact, after the explanation, the patient may be even more insistent in the request for antibiotics. As described by the Symptomatic Cycle framework, when the physician explains that antibiotics will not help the patient and the patient persists in the request, the

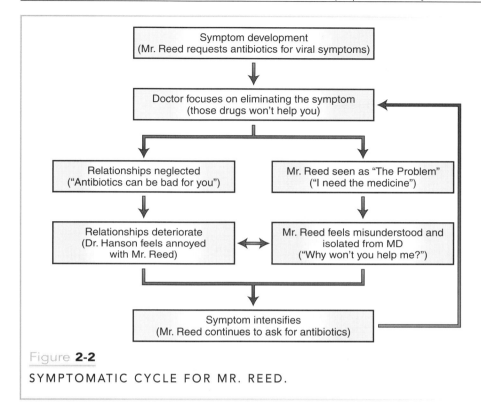

Figure **2-2**

SYMPTOMATIC CYCLE FOR MR. REED.

tendency for the physician is to continue to do more of the same. That is, the physician's tendency is to find other ways to "convince" the patient that antibiotics would not be helpful. This is not a bad approach, *per se*. However, it can be damaging if the physician focuses on changing the patient's mind to the *exclusion* of the doctor-patient relationship. This is what leads to a deterioration in the relationship. The patient may feel misunderstood and isolated, which then further fuels the request for antibiotics.

Analyzing this interaction using the Symptomatic Cycle as a map, the initial presenting concerns are from the cold: runny nose, sore throat, and headache. The focus of the interaction however, quickly turns to the request for antibiotics. This request starts to organize the interaction between the doctor and the patient.

> **Dr. Hanson continues the conversation,** *"It's not that I don't want to help, but I really don't want to hurt you. As I said, antibiotics really don't help cure a cold, despite what a lot of people think."*

> **Mr. Reed pleads his case,** *Well, they have helped me in the past. My old family doctor used to give them to me all the time and they worked. I was up and running in no time."*

> Dr. Hanson, beginning to feel frustrated by the circular nature of the conversation, responds, *"Years ago physicians used to prescribe antibiotics much more frequently than we do today. We have learned a lot about when it's best to prescribe those medicines."*
>
> Mr. Reed sees an opportunity and pounces, *"Exactly my point! It seems to me that this is one of those times."*

This conversation is stuck. The focus on the symptom—the request for antibiotics—has led to an impasse between Mr. Reed and Dr. Hanson. We see how the impasse is generated by Mr. Reed's focus on antibiotics and Dr. Hanson's feeling of powerlessness to change his mind. The problem for Dr. Hanson is that he is starting to feel trapped. On the one hand, if he continues in the circular conversation with Mr. Reed, he will become increasingly frustrated. On the other hand, if he gives in and prescribes the drug, he may feel that he has lowered his professional standards. He may also feel irritated with Mr. Reed and be thinking, "If he would just stop insisting on the drug, this would be fine." What Dr. Hanson needs at this point is a map to guide him through the impasse.

# Traveling Without a Map

At the risk of over-generalizing, allow us to use a common stereotype to illustrate a point. Loading up your loved ones into the family car for a summer vacation can be a risky proposition if you fail to take along a map. This is particularly true when the driver has a strong aversion to asking for directions. A sense of excitement and adventure can quickly transform into frustration and conflict after a few errant left turns. While ultimately, you get where you wanted to go, without a map the trip has been more difficult than it needed to be. (You see where we are going with this.)

In the regular practice of clinical medicine, most physicians use their medical knowledge and interpersonal expertise quite effectively. Most people trust and like their doctor (18-20) and physicians tend to be quite good in dealing with people. However, when physicians depend too heavily on their interpersonal skills, even when they are no longer working, this overdependence may inadvertently contribute to the problem.

As we tell our first-year medical students, being nice is important, but it is not enough; physicians must develop a set of sophisticated techniques for dealing with the difficult encounters that they will inevitably have with their patients. Like on the family vacation, when a physician is faced with the complex and unknown territory of a difficult encounter with a patient, the absence of a map will lead to the same experience as in the family car: conflict.

We have proposed (16) that a common pattern exists in the way physicians try to help patients when there is conflict. As we have seen, unsuccessful attempts to help are followed by an increasing sense of frustration, which can lead to an impasse if the troublesome behavior persists. This frustration leads to withdrawal from the relationship and feelings of anger toward the patient. As the anger increases, a sense of urgency develops around the case followed by feelings of failure by the physician. Finally, the physician blames the patient for the problem and often gives a psychiatric diagnosis ("He's borderline, what do you expect?"). When this happens, both physician and patient end up feeling isolated.

In the case we discussed above, Mr. Reed and Dr. Hanson are locked in an impasse around the issue of prescribing antibiotics for a cold. Using the Symptomatic Cycle as our map, it is easy to see how the relationship with the patient gets neglected as the impasse grows. But what is driving the impasse? In his efforts to feel better, Mr. Reed has become focused on only one solution—having Dr. Hanson prescribe an antibiotic. This suggests inflexibility on the part of Mr. Reed and is usually the result of being cut off from one's own internal resources (21). That is, there are many ways for a person to cope with the distress of cold symptoms—over-the-counter medicines, support from loved ones, self-reassurance, or folk remedies. Perhaps Mr. Reed has tried all of those options but still feels strongly that Dr. Hanson has the answer. Mr. Reed may also have friends and family members reinforcing his narrow view of how to cope ("Have you called the doctor yet?"). As we will see in Chapter 3, the challenge for both the patient and the physician is to work collaboratively in trying to help Mr. Reed cope with having a cold. Dr. Hanson can continue to try and convince Mr. Reed of the uselessness of antibiotics to treat a cold, or increase his own flexibility and change strategies. The Symptomatic Cycle can be a powerful tool for helping physicians change strategies, and in Chapters 5 through 10, we will present concrete examples of how to apply it in clinical practice.

The ultimate goal of using the Symptomatic Cycle as a map is to help physicians think *differently* about their relationships with patients. A different way of thinking can help physicians respond in a new way to the impasse and open the door to a collaborative approach to the  problem. This framework can then help physicians tap their own creative resources by forming a different understanding of the problem. Now let's look at a very different case that is a bit more intense to reinforce how the Symptomatic Cycle can be applied in clinical medicine.

# Drama in the ICU

Jack Andrews is an 83-year-old man with diabetes, a history of heart disease, and some signs of early dementia. He is in the ICU after suffering a catastrophic stroke and requires mechanical ventilation to sustain his life. After several weeks without any improvement, the medical staff have come to view his course of treatment as no longer beneficial and suggest withdrawing life-support. Mr. Andrews had not completed a living will and did not assign a health care proxy, and his wife is deceased. Thus, the decision of whether to remove life support has fallen to his three children. Two of the three children live nearby and have had a good relationship with their father. These two children agree that life support should be withdrawn and their father should be allowed to die. The third child lives two thousand miles away and has a long history of conflict with his father. When he arrives in the ICU, he demands that everything medically possible be done to save his father's life. This child is argumentative with his siblings and the medical staff, accusing all of "giving up on Dad."

Dr. Jamison is Mr. Andrews' intensive care doctor and finds this type of case to be frustrating for several reasons. First, he in no way wants to contribute to Mr. Andrew's suffering; second, medically he does not see any meaningful benefit to continuing mechanical ventilation; and finally, practically speaking, mediating conflicts with upset family members is both time-consuming and stressful. On a typical day in the ICU he cares for 10-15 other patients, but this one case will end up dominating most of the day.

How Dr. Jamison responds to the Andrews family will be key to the eventual outcome of this case. If Jamison believes that the third child is simply a disruption, he may respond in a controlling manner ("Sir, the type of behavior you are demonstrating is not permissible in an ICU. If you continue, we will call security and have you removed from the hospital."). This approach may well lead to an escalation of the conflict between Dr. Jamison and Mr. Andrews' son. If Jamison deals with the disrupting son by avoiding him, this may minimize unpleasant time in the short run, but will likely increase the conflict in the long-term. Without a map to guide interactions with this family, the medical staff can find themselves lost in the wilderness of an impasse.

Using the Symptomatic Cycle as a conceptual framework for the impasse can help Dr. Jamison alter his understanding of what is happening by shifting his thoughts from blaming the son ("He's disruptive and a trouble maker—where has he been for the past decade?") to trying to build a collaborative relationship with him ("He is disruptive, but he must be feeling isolated. I'll start by asking him about his relationship with his father."). Figure 2-3 puts this case in the framework of the Symptomatic Cycle.

The "symptoms" are the son's demand for an aggressive approach to his father's care and his argumentative dealings with family members and staff. He also raises his voice and once punched a soda machine in the ICU family lounge. As the son becomes increasingly demanding, he is seen as "the problem," and the staff focus on getting him to stop being so disruptive. They respond, unintentionally, by being threatening and controlling ("Sir, if you want to see your father, you will have to calm down."). Relationships are thereby neglected and deteriorate further. The paradox in the son's behavior is that the more disruptive he becomes, the more people withdraw from, and try to control, him. This can result in the son feeling isolated and misunderstood, which may increase his disruptive behavior. Dr Jamison's first meeting with the disruptive son shows how staying focused on the symptom escalates disruptive behavior.

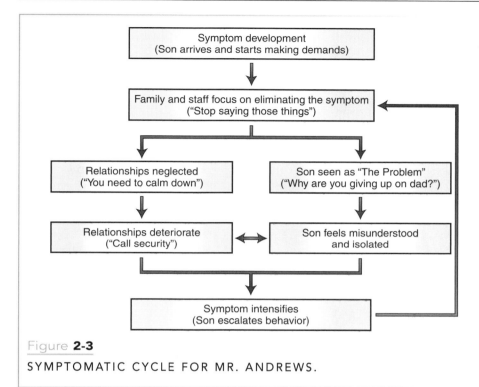

Figure **2-3**

SYMPTOMATIC CYCLE FOR MR. ANDREWS.

**Dr. Jamison begins,** *"Mr. Andrews, I understand that my resident, Dr. Woods, has filled you in on your father's medical condition. Do you have any questions for me?"*

**The son replies a bit sarcastically,** *"Here's what I don't get, Doc—why are you guys giving up on my father? I mean, he just had a stroke, and you're already saying it's time to pull the plug."*

**Dr. Jamison responds with concern and expertise,** *"Mr. Andrews, given the amount of damage in your father's brain from the stroke, we don't see how he could possibly recover in any meaningful way."*

**The son becomes irritated and replies angrily,** *"Let me tell you something about my dad—he wasn't a quitter in his life and he sure as heck wouldn't want a bunch of quitters taking care of him!"*

**Dr. Jamison feels a flash of anger and starts to become controlling,** *"Mr. Andrews, you need to calm down. We're doing our best to help your—"*

**The son raises the stakes, interrupting,** *"You call killing him helping him? I don't know where you went to medical school, but I thought doctors were supposed to save lives, not end them!"*

The impasse has arrived. Dr. Jamison is caught in the cycle of conflict and control. Conflict has taken the form of an escalating disagreement with Mr. Andrews' son. The son's frustration is being expressed toward Dr. Jamison, who in turn tries to assert control by telling the son to calm down. The focus is on the disruptive behavior and not the relationship.

Using the Symptomatic Cycle to understand this problem can help Dr. Jamison to shift away from the symptom (the son's disruptive behavior) and toward the relationship ("Look, we both want what is best for your dad. Let's spend some time talking about your views on that."). "Focusing on the relationship" means that the physician uses the framework of building a relationship as the organizing principle that drives his behavior in the face of an impasse. So instead of being distracted by the son's disruptive behavior and thinking, "He needs to settle down," the physician is focused on how he can build a collaborative relationship with a person who is frustrated and potentially frightened. This framework focuses on the relational aspects of the problem, thus helping the physician to learn what is driving the impasse. Now that Drs. Hanson and Jamison understand what is driving the stalemates they are facing, it is time to move toward resolution. In the next chapter, we will build on these scenarios by introducing the Physician-as-Collaborator Model, which they can use to try to resolve the impasses.

**Summary**

In this chapter we showed that:

- Symptoms are connected to systems.

- The Symptomatic Cycle helps us start with a symptom and broaden our understanding of an impasse to include the system.

- There is value in shifting your focus from the presenting symptom to the relationships.

# References

1. **Minuchin S.** Families and Family Therapy. Cambridge, MA: Harvard University Press; 1974:vii.

2. **Minuchin S, Nichols MP, Lee WY.** Assessing Families and Couples: From Symptom to System. Boston: Pearson; 2007.

3. **Minuchin S, Fishman HC.** Family Therapy Techniques. Cambridge, MA: Harvard University Press; 1981.

4. **Minuchin S, Fishman HC.** Family Therapy Techniques. Cambridge, MA: Harvard University Press; 1981:71-2.

5. **Crouch MA, Roberts L, eds.** The Family in Medical Practice: A Family Systems Primer. New York:Springer-Verlag; 1987.

6. **Brendler J, Silver M, Haber M, Sargent J.** Madness, Chaos, and Violence: Therapy with Families at the Brink. New York: Basic Books; 1991.

7. **Hoffman L.** Beyond power and control: toward a "second order" family systems therapy. Fam Systems Med. 1985;3:381-96.

8. **Micucci JA.** The Adolescent in Family Therapy: Breaking the Cycle of Conflict and Control. New York: The Guilford Press; 1998.

9. **McDaniel SH, Hepworth J, Doherty WJ.** Medical Family Therapy: A Biopsychosocial Approach to Families with Health Problems. New York: Basic Books; 1992.

10. **Rolland JS.** Families, Illness, and Disability: An Integrative Treatment Model. New York: Basic Books; 1994.

11. **Kazak A.** Pediatric psychosocial preventive health model (PPPHM): research, practice, and collaboration in pediatric family systems medicine. Fam Systems Health. 2006;24:381-95.

12. **Kazak A, Rourke M, Crump T.** Families and other systems in pediatric psychology. In: Roberts M, ed. Handbook of Pediatric Psychology, 3rd ed. New York: The Guilford Press; 2003:159-75.

13. **Kazak A, Simms S, Rourke M.** Family systems practice in pediatric psychology. J Pediatr Psychol. 2002;27:133-43.

14. **Kazak A, Blackall GF, Himelstein B, et al.** Producing systemic change in pediatric practice: an intervention protocol for reducing distress during painful procedures. Fam Systems Med. 1995;13:173-85.

15. **Blackall GF, Simms S.** Resolving therapeutic impasses in medical settings: a case study. Fam Systems Health. 2002;20:253-64.

16. **Blackall GF, Green MJ, Simms S.** Application of systems principles to resolving ethical dilemmas in medicine. J Clin Ethics. 2005;16:20-28.

17. **Micucci JA.** The Adolescent in Family Therapy: Breaking the Cycle of Conflict and Control. New York: The Guilford Press; 1998:18.

18. **Door-Goold S.** Trust, distrust and trustworthiness. J Gen Intern Med. 2002;17:79-81.

19. **Kao AC, Green DC, Davis NA, et al.** Patients' trust in their physicians: effects of choice, continuity, and payment method. J Gen Intern Med. 1998;13:681-6.

20. **Pearson SD, Reake LH.** Patients' trust in physicians: many theories, few measures, and little data. J Gen Intern Med. 2000;15:509-13.

21. **Simms S.** A protocol for seriously ill children with severe psychosocial symptoms: avoiding potential disasters. Fam Systems Med. 1995;13:245-57.

# Chapter 3
# How to Begin: Building Collaborative Relationships

All of the physicians who have been introduced thus far are looking for guidance on how to proceed with their patients. The Symptomatic Cycle helps explain how the impasses they experienced have come to be. The next goal is to figure out how to approach, and hopefully resolve, these impasses. To accomplish this, it is time to shift from the Physician-as-Expert Model to the Physician-as-Collaborator Model. In explaining the Physician-as-Collaborator Model, we will introduce Five Universal Principles that will provide concrete guidance on how to develop collaborative relationships with your patients.

**Key Terms**

- Physician-as-Collaborator Model
- Five Universal Principles for a Collaborative Doctor-Patient Relationship
- ARCH

# Physician-As-Collaborator Model

The concept of doctors and patients working together, or collaborating, is not new. Previous authors have articulated models of "shared decision making" that include at least two people being involved in a process where both parties participate, information is exchanged, and agreement is ultimately reached on how to proceed (1-5). This approach to practicing medicine is important because it demonstrates respect for the individual, it helps patients to become more engaged in decisions about their health, it encourages individuals to take responsibility for their health and well-being, and it takes some of the burden of decision making away from the physician. While physicians may well recognize the importance of working together with their patients, they may not know *how* to be collaborative in the face of a serious impasse. This is where we help.

The overarching premise of the Physician-as-Collaborator Model is that the patient and doctor are partners in a therapeutic relationship, and decisions are made in a collaborative fashion. Each partner brings expertise to the relationship, and both types of expertise are equally valuable and necessary to build a collaborative relationship. The patient is an expert at defining treatment goals and objectives in terms of their own values and preferences. The physician is an expert in using medical knowledge and skills to help achieve the goals articulated by the patient. The Physician-as-Collaborator Model brings the expertise of both parties together and works in conjunction with the Physician-as-Expert Model. Figure 3-1 illustrates how these two styles compliment each other.

The Physician-as-Expert Model is commonly used and familiar to both doctors and patients. However, even though the main reason people go to the doctor is for medical expertise, the Model's usefulness is limited when medical expertise is not enough to prevent or resolve an impasse. In contrast, the goal of the Physician-as-Collaborator Model is to avoid or resolve an impasse with a patient by keeping the doctor and patient engaged in a collaborative relationship even in the face of an unremitting medical or behavioral problem. By keeping the doctor and patient in a collaborative mode, it prevents both parties from becoming ensnared in an escalating conflict that results in emotional withdrawal from the relationship. As we saw in Chapter Two, emotional withdrawal is what feeds the impasse and keeps the Symptomatic Cycle alive.

The first step in the Physician-as-Collaborator Model is for the physician to attend to and monitor relevant medical problems. Even when it appears that the patient has received an extensive work-up with negative findings, the inherent uncertainty that is part of practicing medicine requires a physician to continually monitor, and reconsider, persistent medical problems. This also reassures the patient that their concerns are being taken seriously.

A second component to the Physician-as-Collaborator Model is for the physician to encourage the patient and family to turn to each other to seek creative ways to cope with distressing symptoms. The physician remains in a

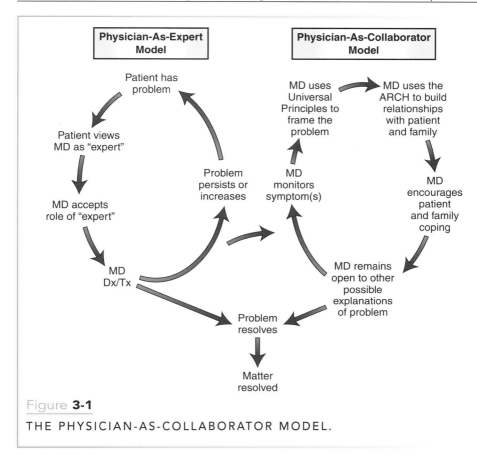

Figure **3-1**

THE PHYSICIAN-AS-COLLABORATOR MODEL.

collaborative mode by partnering with the patient and family in their efforts to cope, while he or she continues to monitor the troubling medical problem.

The third component of the Physician-as-Collaborator Model is for the physician to remain open to other possible explanations of the problem. A key part of facilitating a collaborative relationship is for the physician to remain flexible in his or her approach to the problem as new information becomes available. This includes seeking out and embracing the patient's expertise regarding their goals, values, and preferences.

On the surface it looks relatively simple to shift from expert to collaborator, even in difficult cases. But if it is so simple, why do good physicians get caught in unproductive cycles of frustration with their patients? Because *while the motivating forces that introduce, and fuel, the cycle are based upon the best of intentions* (the patient wants to get better and the physician wants to help), the efforts to resolve the impasse are misguided. As we will see in later cases, as the cycle escalates it leaves the patient feeling abandoned and the physician struggling with feelings of failure.

---

Box **3-1**

# Five Universal Principles for a Collaborative Doctor-Patient Relationship

1. **Competence:** All patients (and families) bring a pre-existing set of competencies to the illness experience.

2. **Connection:** Isolation and disconnection from important relationships exacerbates psychological distress.

3. **Control:** Control is a myth.

4. **Contribution:** Your blind spots fuel impasses. See your role in, or contribution to, the impasse.

5. **Collaboration:** All of the above principles apply to medical staff as well as patients and families.

---

We have developed a system of five universal principles (6,7) that can be used as practical tools for physicians to develop a collaborative relationship and, when necessary, resolve impasses with patients and their families. You might think about these universal principles as the 5 C's (Box 3-1).

## *Principle #1. Competence: All Patients (and Families) Bring a Pre-Existing Set of Competencies to the Illness Experience*

This is the most important principle in this chapter. For our purposes, "competencies" refers to the things in life over which people have a sense of mastery. The key competencies are derived from one's primary roles in life. An attending physician may feel competent in her ability to diagnose and treat common illnesses in her specialty. A mechanic may feel a sense of competence about repairing cars. A patient may feel a sense of competence as a mother and wife.

When faced with stress, an individual may lack a feeling of competence or mastery over the stressful event. For example, recalling the experience of sitting in your first medical school lecture may bring back memories of anxiety or uncertainty. As a new student, you may have felt insignificant or small. While you no doubt possessed the essential skills to be a successful medical student (the ability to stay focused, study, and learn) you had not yet mastered the material necessary to judge your own competence. With hard work, persistence, and the help of teachers and mentors, you gradually learned how to succeed as a medical student, and the anxiety likely faded. For patients who are untried at being ill, the experience can be similar.

When illness hits, patients typically feel vulnerable. They do not know what to expect or how to behave. They see the physician as someone who can help them feel more secure and, with this security, they hope to gain an increased sense of competence. This increased sense of competence enables the patient to explore different ways of thinking about their health problem. When people feel competent, they can cope more effectively by being more open and flexible in response to stressors. For example, a patient with newly diagnosed Type II diabetes may be concerned about the finger sticks required for daily glucose monitoring. He may report being needle phobic and be worried that he will not be able to successfully monitor his glucose level. With encouragement from his physician to be persistent, in a few weeks, and after repeated practice, the patient exhibits competence in reporting that the finger sticks are no problem.

## *Key Task for Principle #1: Highlight Competencies*

Recognizing that everyone has competencies is an important first step in developing a collaborative relationship and overcoming an impasse with a patient. By highlighting competencies, one shifts the focus away from what someone *cannot* do to what he or she *can* do. This helps reinforce pre-existing strengths rather than focusing on deficiencies.

In Chapter Two we introduced Mr. Reed, the patient with a cold who insisted that Dr. Hanson give him a prescription for antibiotics. We used the Symptomatic Cycle to highlight the circular nature of the interaction. The more that Dr. Hanson tried to explain that antibiotics would not cure a cold, the more Mr. Reed wanted the prescription. Mr. Reed's approach to coping with the cold had become rigid, meaning he saw only one solution to his problem. The lack of flexibility suggests that Mr. Reed may have lost sight of some of his other competencies. He may be consumed by the discomfort of his symptoms or he may be highly influenced by those around him (like a relative or friend saying "You need to be on antibiotics."). Whatever the cause, Dr. Hanson and Mr. Reed are locked in an impasse.

A key part of overcoming this impasse is for Dr. Hanson to be aware of his own beliefs about his patient. If Dr. Hanson believes that Mr. Reed is obstinate and narrow-minded, it is going to be hard to develop a collaborative relationship and focus on Mr. Reed's competencies. This contrasts with Dr. Hanson believing that Mr. Reed is suffering and has lost sight of his innate competencies. This change in beliefs will alter how he approaches Mr. Reed. Here is how Dr. Hanson highlighted Mr. Reed's competencies in an attempt to overcome the impasse:

> *"Mr. Reed, I know you are very uncomfortable right now and it is hard to cope with feeling so lousy. I also know that in the past you have figured out ways to tolerate physical discomfort and corral your worries. I believe you can do this again. What do you think?"*

> **Mr. Reed pauses thoughtfully and responds,** *"I have sometimes, yes, that's true. But this time it's much worse. I don't*

*see how I am going to get better without any antibiotics. It's
not as though I haven't already been trying to put up with
this."*

**Dr. Hanson continues to highlight Mr. Reed's competen-
cies,** *"I understand that you are trying hard to cope with
this."*

**Mr. Reed connects positively to Dr. Hanson's comment by
responding,** *"I have, and it's no picnic. Let me tell you, when
you go night after night without sleep, it gets to you."*

**Dr. Hanson realizes that the tone of the conversation is
shifting and pursues his strategy,** *"Of course it does, and I
admire how much you have already put up with. On the
other hand, I believe that you will get better. I guess what I
am asking of you is to try to wait this thing out. Will you give
my idea 48 hours?"*

**Mr. Reed hesitates and voices concern,** *"I don't know if I
can. What if I get worse?"*

Mr. Reed is concerned that he will be left alone with his suffering and that
he may feel worse. Dr. Hanson's efforts at highlighting Mr. Reed's competencies have been helpful, but he needs to reassure Mr. Reed that he is not withdrawing from the relationship.

*"If you get worse, or if there is a side of you that doubts what
I say, then call me and I will see you. Then we can reassess
what is happening."*

By pointing out that he has been able to tolerate physical discomfort in the
past, Dr. Hanson highlights Mr. Reed's competencies. He stays connected to
Mr. Reed by offering to see him if his symptoms get worse. While this may
seem simple, it successfully shifts the conversation away from the impasse
while reinforcing Mr. Reed's strengths. Furthermore, by offering to meet with
him if his symptoms get worse, Dr. Hanson is sending the message that he
will continue to work with Mr. Reed. A key part of breaking an impasse is to
focus on relationships, and the offer to be available to Mr. Reed is a way to
do this.

In this example, Dr. Hanson chose to highlight a competency related to Mr.
Reed's ability to tolerate discomfort in the past. There are times, however,
when a physician may not be aware of a patient's medical competencies. It is
strategically important, therefore, to get to know a person and be able to build
a bridge from areas of their life where they are competent to the medical problem being faced. To further underscore how to build a bridge from a patient's
life to their medical problems, consider the following case.

One of us once consulted with a 12-year-old boy who had recently been diagnosed with non-Hodgkin's lymphoma. The reason for the consult was that

the boy was crying constantly and had withdrawn from important relationships. In the initial meeting, the child was sad and looked defeated. When asked to talk about things he used to do prior to being diagnosed with cancer, the boy slowly started talking about how he was an outstanding football player. He was then asked where the football player had gone? This question reminded the child that he had positive qualities that he could use in his fight with cancer. After a few minutes, the boy said it was time to find the football player.

Patients bring competencies from all parts of their lives that can be helpful in coping with medical adversity. One contribution a physician can make to developing a collaborative relationship and resolving an impasse is to build a bridge from the boardroom, the playroom, the classroom, or a locker room to the exam room in a way that reminds people of their abilities to cope with adversity.

## Principle #2. Connection: Isolation and Disconnection From Important Relationships Exacerbates Psychological Distress

When people are cut off from others in the face of adversity, they become frightened and find ways to express that fear. While some people connect to others in a crisis, others express their distress in a way that paradoxically drives people away, leaving them further isolated.

## Key Task for Principle #2: Focus on Relationships

Focusing on relationships is how people decrease isolation and disconnection. By initiating authentic and non-manipulative contact, the physician can use her commitment to the relationship to promote change. This principle can be applied in the case of Mr. Andrews.

### Back to the ICU

Fred Andrews, the son of the 83-year-old man who had suffered a devastating stroke, disagreed that it was time to withdraw life support and let his father die. He accused Dr. Jamison and his staff of being quitters. As Mr. Andrews' behavior escalated, the medical staff focused more on his behavior and less on their relationship with him. As a result, Mr. Andrews became increasingly cut off from the other people involved in the conflict.

The Symptomatic Cycle provides the framework for how to understand this case. According to the Symptomatic Cycle, the more the medical staff tries to change Mr. Andrews' behavior, the more his behavior will escalate because attempts to get him to calm down are likely to be experienced as controlling. But if Dr. Jamison alters his attitude about Mr. Andrews, viewing him not as an out-of-town trouble-maker, but rather as an isolated and disconnected individual who cares about his father, this will help him to build a collaborative relationship with this troubled son. Dr. Jamison tried to shift the emphasis away from the troubling behavior and toward the relationship by highlighting Mr. Andrews' competencies as a son:

> "I can see that you are fighting hard for your dad's interests. I can also see that there is disagreement among you, your siblings, and the medical staff. I believe this is very important, and I wonder if we can talk for a while about why you feel so strongly that we should continue aggressive medical care for your dad."

This approach sends a clear message that Dr. Jamison will not attempt to control the son with threats or abandonment. It is also a direct attempt to reduce Mr. Andrews' isolation by offering to spend time with him and to listen to his point of view. This will also help Mr. Andrews to feel included in the medical decision-making process. The goal here is not to get him to change his mind. The goal is to build a collaborative relationship that will enhance Dr. Jamison's understanding of Mr. Andrews. The deeper understanding will help Dr. Jamison access his own creativity in an effort to resolve the impasse. The conversation continues with Mr. Andrews being skeptical.

> "Doctor Jamison, I appreciate you wanting to hear my side of this. But if you think you're going to change my mind using this psychobabble stuff, it's not going to happen."

> **Dr. Jamison tries to be explicit about his motives, replying,** "I am not trying to change your mind. Only you can do that. Right now, I really don't understand why you feel so strongly about this. It would help me if I knew more."

> **Mr. Andrews starts to open up,** "You have to understand that my dad and I had our problems. You might say we were too much alike to get along. Even though we had our share of spats, I understood the man. He never gave up on anything in life. That's just not how he lived."

> **Dr. Jamison, continuing to highlight Mr. Andrews' competence as a son,** "This is very helpful. I didn't know your father before his stroke. I think I'm starting to understand that even though there was distance between the two of you, both geographically and emotionally, there was still an important connection."

> **Mr. Andrews responds with surprising honesty,** "Darn straight there was. And I don't think it's right for my brother and sister and you folks here to think you know what he would have wanted."

**Jamison holds the course,** *"I can tell you want to do right by your father at this critical time. What do you think we should do next?"*

**Andrews replies,** *"I'm not sure, but I don't think we should pull the plug."*

**Jamison senses a shift in his relationship with Mr. Andrews,** *"I agree; it's not time. But I would like you to promise me that even though we may disagree, we will continue to talk."*

*"Done."*

Dr. Jamison has shifted the focus entirely away from the son's behavior by building his relationship with him. As he begins to focus on the son's relationship with his father, the son starts to relax. Dr. Jamison's search for the son's competencies has facilitated a shift in their conversation from antagonistic to collaborative. While the case is still in limbo, progress is being made. The Symptomatic Cycle has been disrupted and the tone of the conversation has become constructive. By asking the son what he thinks should happen next, Dr. Jamison has attempted to give Mr. Andrews some control, an issue that is at the heart of the third universal principle.

## *Principle #3. Control: Control Is a Myth*

Interpersonally, control involves power and acquiescence. When one person has control over another, he or she has power. The power comes not from the "control" *per se*, but from the other person's decision to acquiesce. Thus, the Physician-as-Expert Model we presented in Chapter One works well when the patient accepts the physician in the role of expert and agrees to follow his or her lead. The physician's control comes from the patient's trust and agreement to do as he or she recommends. Without the acquiescence, there is no control. But, therein lies the paradox. If a physician believes that he or she has control in a relationship with a patient he or she may unintentionally and inadvertently contribute to a conflict by acting in a controlling fashion.

For example, making unilateral decisions, even when one firmly believes it is in the patient's best interest, can be experienced by some patients as controlling. There are, of course, times in clinical medicine when unilateral decision making is appropriate. For instance, during medical emergencies patients are usually quite comfortable with the doctor making the decisions. However, what we are addressing here are situations where the patient is *not* comfortable with the doctor taking charge in this way.

The decision not to prescribe an antibiotic for a patient who has a cold can be accepted by some patients as appropriate. There is an unspoken contract between the doctor and the patient where most patients decide to accept the Physician-as-Expert Model and respect the physician's decision. Other patients, like Mr. Reed, push back. They disagree with the physician and decide to express their disagreement. This sets off a power struggle between the doctor and patient. Once this power struggle starts, the physician can continue to act in the role of Physician-as-Expert or try to disengage from the power struggle. Staying engaged in the power struggle will escalate the conflict. So how does one avoid or disengage from a power struggle with a patient?

## Key Task for Principle #3: Move from Control to Collaboration

The first step in avoiding or disengaging from a power struggle is to acknowledge that control is a myth. This is done by avoiding unilateral decision-making and working toward a collaborative problem-solving process. Such a process involves the following guidelines.

1. **Acknowledge that you are not solely responsible for the patient's outcome.** For example, you can prescribe all of the exercise and medications in the world for an obese, diabetic, hypertensive patient with chronic back pain but he will not get better until he makes a decision to change his lifestyle.

2. **Identify your role, limits, and function.** Know what you can do. Know what you cannot do. Know what you are willing to do.

3. **Focus on the controllable.** You cannot control the patient's behavior, but you can control your response to a patient. For instance, in the case of the diabetic, obese patient mentioned above, focusing on what you can control (making sound medical and lifestyle recommendations, staying connected to your patient) can help alleviate the frustration of seeing your patient continue to suffer and plead for help. So, instead of taking a controlling stance ("Sir, you must lose weight!"), you can take a collaborative approach that incorporates the previously mentioned guidelines. Saying, "Sir, if you do the things I recommend, I believe you will start to feel better. If you don't, then you will continue to feel this way and perhaps even worse. I am happy to be your doctor, but in order for you to feel better, we both have to contribute," will keep you focused on your response and not your patient's behavior.

The scenario of Mr. Reed's requests for antibiotics illustrates these concepts. In the last conversation between Mr. Reed and his physician, Dr. Hanson was trying to move the conversation away from the conflict by focusing on Mr. Reed's competencies. The proposal was for Mr. Reed to wait 48 hours to see if his cold symptoms improved. The next day Mr. Reed called Hanson's office and asked to be seen again:

*"Doctor Hanson, I'm getting worse. My cough is keeping me up, I'm exhausted, and I can't sleep. I need the medicine."*

Sticking to his strategy of highlighting Mr. Reed's competencies while being collaborative, Dr. Hanson responds: *"I'm glad you've tried to cope with your discomfort. I'm also glad you felt comfortable calling me today. So the problem is what to do. I still feel that an antibiotic is not appropriate. However, I also understand that you are really uncomfortable and concerned about your health. Here are the things to look out for that might suggest that this is more than a viral infection: high fever, chills, coughing up yellow or green sputum, pain in your ears or sinuses, or if it hurts when you take a deep breath. If any of those things occur, please call me right away."*

Mr. Reed reluctantly agrees, *"OK, but what if none of those things happens and I still feel this bad?"*

Maintaining a collaborative stance, Dr. Hanson replies, *"Well, I would be happy to see you again if you are no better in two days. Also, I would be willing to call in one of my colleagues and get his input."*

In this exchange, Dr. Hanson avoided a power struggle by using the Physician-as-Collaborator Model. Even through disagreement, he attended to his relationship with his patient. He knew his role, limits, and function and he was willing to collaboratively set a limit. He avoided asserting control in the form of unilateral decision-making ("Mr. Reed, how many times do I have to tell you I won't prescribe an antibiotic?") and established a collaborative tone to the conversation ("Here is what to look out for. Call me anytime. We can seek input from one of my colleagues."). The important point here is not whether the doctor and patient continue to disagree, but that the doctor is open and honest with his patient and gives the patient an opportunity to do the same. Not all cases work out the way we want them to. We cannot control all outcomes. But what we can control is the way we understand and respond to impasses with patients. A key part of effectively responding to these impasses is to be aware of our blind spots, which is the fourth principle.

## *Principle #4. Contribution: Your Blind Spots Fuel Impasses*

For the purposes of this book, blind spots refer to instances when one fails to see his or her role in, or contribution to, a conflict or impasse. Our beliefs sometimes become our blind spots. Believing that the "doctor always knows best" or that children do not need to have a say in their healthcare decisions are examples of blind spots. Rigidly clinging to such beliefs contributes to the impasse.

As part of writing this book, we interviewed physicians in three different focus groups about the types of clinical encounters they found particularly

challenging. The following statement illustrates one physician's blind spot—
the role his isolation and disconnection played in conflicts with his "difficult"
patients:

> *"I don't routinely check my schedule the night before clinic
> anymore. I don't want to lose sleep. I call it the cringe factor.
> I see someone's name on the schedule and I say to myself:'
> Whoa! I can't believe that patient is here again!' I take a
> deep breath and get ready for the encounter."*

This is an example of a physician who is struggling to gain a sense of competence over the demands certain patients place on him. It also illustrates
how his dread has resulted in his becoming isolated and disconnected from
certain parts of himself. These comments were made by a highly skilled and
respected physician. He is a creative and deeply intellectual person. Yet, the
same skills he routinely applies to complex clinical problems do not help him
in a difficult interpersonal encounter with a patient. He views the encounter
as something to be avoided until the last moment, as opposed to being intrigued by the highly complex interaction. This is out of character for this person. He embraces, even thrives, on difficult medical cases. He is intrigued by
complex issues. Yet those same skills are absent when it comes to dealing
with patients that tax his interpersonal skills. He goes on to speak of patients
who seek narcotics:

> *"I feel an obligation to them because I'm an ultra-specialist
> in that particular disease. They are my patients, and in many
> cases patients I've known for a long time. They would not
> want to see another physician, and I would not want them to
> see another physician. In a sense, they're stuck with me and
> I'm stuck with them. They have reasons why they continue to
> see me and I have reasons why I want to continue to see
> them. I'm their doctor so I can't give them up. On the other
> hand, I guess part of my personality is that I'm a pushover.
> They'll tell me a story and while I should put up a wall and
> say no, in most circumstances I'm going to give in and give
> them what they want. I'm not necessarily feeling so good
> about it."*

The bind for the physician is that he wants to "be there" for his patient, yet
at some level, he feels exploited by the encounter. As a result, he avoids the
interaction as long as possible, then enters the room with the sole purpose of
getting out unscathed. It is easy to see how the relationship with his patient
gets neglected, which in turn creates distress. He continues with his story.

> *"It's frustrating because I'm sitting there waiting for that part
> of the encounter to take place, dreading it because it always
> comes up. I don't quite trust them. They know I don't quite
> trust them. They're going to do their best to get what they*

*feel they need or want from me. We both know it's coming and it's uncomfortable. It's much easier when you have no emotional or professional relationship with them. They come to see you once and they ask for pain meds; that's easy—I don't know you, I'm not going to give you pain med-icine. But it's more complex when we have an investment in people."*

The physician describes a process where he feels medically competent, he knows he should not give the medicines, but he lacks a sense of competence on how to work collaboratively with the patient in areas where they disagree. In the end, he gives in and then feels bad about himself.

## Key Task for Principle #4: See Your Role in, or Contribution to, the Impasse

The struggle for this physician was interpersonal, not medical, and his chal-lenge is to develop competence in dealing with the interpersonal aspects of these difficult patient encounters. But first, he needs to see his blind spots— how *he* contributes to the conflict. His current strategy is to avoid the en-counter until the last minute, then do his best to get in and out as quickly as possible. That avoidance is his blind spot. The lack of competence drives avoidance, which in turn creates distance with his patient. This is the with-drawal we presented in the Physician-as-Expert Model in Chapter One and is what prevents him from operating in the Physician-as-Collaborator Model. The net result is conflict with his patient.

Another physician described a scenario where he, too, struggled:

*"This was a new consult that came to me. She reported cog-nitive and gait dysfunction. She very quickly she told me that she had seen a rheumatologist but was no longer seeing this person because "He's a moron." She also saw a neurologist, but unfortunately he was a moron, too, so she couldn't see him anymore. She had heard how 'brilliant' I was. Within a couple of weeks [she had made] multiple phone calls ex-pressing her displeasure with me, and within four months she was moving on because I was the moron. Cases like that certainly provide some frustration."*

This physician saw the writing on the wall but felt powerless to change the outcome. As we pointed out earlier, control is a myth. In this case, the physi-cian clearly lacked control over the outcome. Among the key tasks we previ-ously delineated in the face of no control was knowing your role, limits, and function. The blind spot in this case was that the physician knew his limits before he took the case, yet he agreed to try to help the patient anyway. His actions were based on the best of intentions—he really wanted to help. But he did not know how to approach the patient in a way that would have either saved him a lot of work by having the patient fire him early, or potentially guide the patient to mental health care. As a result, he went from medical genius to moron.

What could the physician have done differently? Since he knew he was unlikely to be able to help this patient, he could have refused to take the case. In medicine, refusing to take a case is bold decision. After all, this patient was in need of help. What kind of physician turns away patients who need help? But there is a difference between turning away a patient in need of help when you have the skills to offer at least some assistance, versus turning away a patient in need when you do not have the appropriate skills. Turning away a patient in need when the physician lacks the necessary skills is part of being an expert. When a CT surgeon refers a patient with chronic headaches to a neurologist, it is considered sound medical practice. Yet finding a way to refer the above patient to a psychologist or a psychiatrist is difficult because of the social stigma associated with mental illness and the fact that certainty in medicine is elusive. There is always the possibility that something medical may indeed have been missed so it is essential to find a way to stay connected to the patient after the mental health referral has been made (we discuss the topic of mental health referrals in Chapter 10).

Another possibility in this scenario is to accept the case and establish a collaborative relationship from the outset, but with explicit expectations about the outcome. A seasoned clinician may see this case and believe that it is highly unlikely that he or she will be able to do anything more than all of the previous physicians who tried to help this patient, but may still feel compelled to take the case. Here is how a physician might approach this patient with the goals of offering a collaborative relationship and reducing one's blind spots:

> *"Mrs. Lyons, I am willing to work with you. But before we decide to work together I need to be clear about expectations. I will do my best to find out what is causing your discomfort, but I don't think it is likely that I will find anything different or better than all of the other doctors you have already seen. That said, I am willing to see you and be part of your struggle with this problem."*

By being explicit from the outset, and presenting a collaborative framework, the physician avoids the trap of feeling compelled to do more of the same, all the while believing that the outcome will be unchanged.

## Principle #5. Collaboration: All of the Above Principles Apply to Medical Staff As Well As Patients and Families

A key part of disrupting destructive patterns of interaction among medical staff, patients, and families is to avoid the urge to put the full burden of change on the patient and family. Medical staff can lead the process of change by viewing themselves as a key part of the resolution of the conflict.

## Key Task for Principle #5: Use Your Experience to Appreciate the Patient's Experience

Your feelings and experience of a difficult encounter with a patient and family can be used as a barometer of the experience for all involved parties. Being self-aware can give you insight into some of the potentially difficult feelings of your patient. Acknowledging your own difficult feelings will then enable you to focus on controlling yourself, rather than on controlling others, which will help you to understand and accept others even when both parties are having difficult feelings (Box 3-2).

---

Box **3-2**

# ARCH: A Great Impasse Prevention Tool

ARCH stands for *Acceptance, Respect, Curiosity* and *Honesty (ARCH)* (see Reference 8). These basic concepts can be integrated into the application of all of the universal principles.

### Acceptance

Acceptance is a challenging task for physicians. It is easy to accept patients when they adore and compliment your extraordinary healing abilities as a physician. However, when patients or family members are angry, demanding, or threatening, it is much more difficult to tolerate, and therefore accept, their behavior. Acceptance does not mean agreement. Rather, it means the physician allows a person to have their feelings, even though you may not like the feelings that person is expressing. The goal of acceptance is for the physician to stop trying to get the patient to change those feelings.

### Respect

Treating people with *respect* sets the groundwork for a collaborative relationship. Respect means listening to the patient, validating his or her concerns, and taking what the patient has to say seriously. Without respect, collaboration is not possible.

### Curiosity

*Curiosity* is the key that unlocks competencies within people. Asking the simple question: "What would a curious person do in this situation?" sets the stage for the physician to migrate away from controlling behaviors ("Sir, if you don't calm down, we will have to call security and have you removed from the hospital.") to curious ones ("Sir, I can see that you are upset. What is it about this situation that is most distressing to you?"). Curious people ask questions like: "What are you most concerned about?" "What is that like for you?" "Can you tell me more about that?" "How do other people in your family view this problem?" "How can I be helpful to you?"

### Honesty

*Honesty* involves a physician recognizing and acknowledging his or her own reactions and feelings in a productive manner with a patient. Honesty includes being honest with yourself as well as your patient. As we saw earlier, having negative feelings toward some patients is a normal part of being human. The key is to use those feelings in a way that promotes a collaborative relationship with your patient. Saying "I find this situation frustrating too. How do you think we can move toward finding a solution?" is an effective way to be honest and collaborative.

Table **3-1**

# Universal Principles and Key Tasks for Approaching Impasses with Patients

| Universal Principle | Key Tasks |
|---|---|
| **Competence:** Patients and families bring competencies to the illness experience | Highlight competencies |
| **Connection:** Isolation and disconnection exacerbates psychological distress | Focus on relationships |
| **Control:** Control is a myth | Move from control to collaboration |
| **Contribution:** Your blind spots fuel impasses | See your role in, or contribution to, the impasse |
| **Collaboration:** All of the above apply to staff as well as patients and families | Use your experience to appreciate the patient's experience |

**Summary**

In this chapter we presented the Physician-as-Collaborator Model and Five Universal Principles to help guide physicians through the complex terrain of impasses with patients. Highlighting competencies, focusing on relationships, moving from control to curiosity, seeing your role in the conflict, and using your experience to appreciate the patient's experience are the principles that will drive the remainder of this book.

One of the Universal Principles we presented was Contribution (Table 3-1); that is, knowing your role or contribution to an impasse. To help you minimize your contribution to an impasse and to maximize your ability to prevent impasses, in Chapter Four we will present some basic skills for communicating with patients.

# References

1. **Charles C, Gafni A, Whelan T.** Shared decision making in the medical encounter: what does it mean? (Or it takes two to tango). Soc Sci Med. 1997;44:681-92.

2. **Makoul G, Clayman ML.** An integrative model of shared decision making in medical encounters. Patient Educ Counsel. 2006;60:301-12.

3. **Maudsley RF, Wilson DR, Neufeld VR, et al.** Educating future physicians for Ontario: Phase II. Acad Med. 2000;75:113-26.

4. **Tuckett D, Boulton M, Olson C. Williams A.** Meetings Between Experts: An Approach to Sharing Ideas in Medical Consultations. London: Tavistock Publications; 1985.

5. **Siegler M.** Searching for moral certainty in medicine: a proposal for a new model of the doctor-patient encounter. Bull N Y Acad Med. 1981;1:56-69.

6. **Blackall GF, Green MJ, Simms S.** Application of systems principles to resolving ethical dilemmas in medicine. J Clin Ethics. 2005;1:20-8.

7. **Simms SG.** A protocol for seriously ill children with severe psychosocial symptoms: avoiding potential disasters. Fam Systems Med. 1995;13:245-57.

8. **Micucci JA.** The Adolescent in Family Therapy: Breaking the Cycle of Conflict and Control. New York: The Guilford Press; 1998:5.

# Chapter 4

# An Ounce of Prevention: How to Avoid Impasses with Patients and Their Families

In clinical medicine, physicians face a wide range of potential problems in the doctor-patient relationship. To help avoid impasses with patients, we will present several straightforward and basic tools that can be used to build strong collaborative relationships between doctors and patients. While it is impossible to completely avoid all impasses, attending to the relationship with your

**Key Terms**
- Back to basics
- Listening
- Let the patient tell their story
- Do I understand?
- Watch your language
- Feelings
- The sounds of silence
- Staying connected

patient when the winds of conflict start to blow will help to avert or curtail problems.

# Back to Basics

In the course of medical training, you were taught basic communication skills for interacting with patients. Sometimes, preventing problems with patients is as simple as relying on these basic techniques. Many of those techniques stress the importance of building a good working relationship with your patient. Family therapists call this "joining" (1). Various books on communication in medicine refer to this as building the relationship (2,3), building rapport (4), and preparing for listening (5). The term is less important than the process. Consider the following two examples, which show different ways to initiate a patient encounter.

## *Scenario #1*

It is an extremely busy day in the outpatient medicine clinic. The attending physician is feeling increasingly frustrated as he gets further behind. He looks at the chart of his next patient as he is about to enter the room and sees that she is a middle-aged woman with what appear to be symptoms of a common cold. He enters the exam room without knocking on the door. He is reading the chart as he enters the room and says:

> *"So, what seems to be the problem today?"*

> **The patient appears to freeze and says,** *"I have a bad cold."*

## *Scenario #2*

It is an extremely busy day in the outpatient medicine clinic. The attending physician is feeling increasingly frustrated as he gets further behind. He glances at the chart of his next patient and sees that she is a middle-aged woman with what appear to be symptoms of a common cold. The physician takes 10 seconds to gather himself before he enters the exam room. He knocks on the door and asks if he can come in. He then enters the room, washes his hands, and introduces himself as he extends his hand. He sits down and says to the patient

> *"So, Mrs. Robbins, how are you today?"*

> **The patient looks at the physician and replies:** *"I'm fine,"* **and then bursts into tears.**

Hopefully, it is evident that Scenario #2 is a more effective way to build a trusting and collaborative relationship with a patient. In this scenario, the physician took a few easy steps to start to build a relationship with his patient. Doing so is not difficult and involves several simple tasks.

1. **The 10-second rule. Take 10 seconds to breathe before you enter the room.** Focusing on your breathing will help your body to relax and your mind to be clear.

2. **Create a warm and inviting atmosphere for the patient.** Introduce yourself, wash your hands, shake hands, and sit down if at all possible when speaking to the patient. Robert Buckman refers to this as getting the physical context right (5).

3. **Be personal.** Use the person's name, look them in the eye, and ask them how they would like to be addressed. On rounds, the patient may be a 37-year-old Caucasian female with aplastic anemia, but to her family, she is Sarah, a caring wife, and mother of three children who is scared silly because she has a bad blood disorder.

4. **Address and listen to everyone in the room.** Many patients will have a family member or friend with them for support. People have a need to be acknowledged and heard, even if they are not the patient.

# Listening

Most doctors believe that they are good listeners, and that they give their patients ample attention. And yet findings from several studies indicate the following:

- The mean time before doctors interrupt their patients is 18-23 seconds (6,10).

- Doctors and patients do not agree on the main presenting problem 50% of the time (7).

- During the doctor-patient encounter, 45% of patients' concerns and 54% of their complaints were not obtained (8).

If we are all such good listeners, how could this be? See Box 4-1.

---

Box **4-1**

## How to Listen

1. Be patient—let your patient tell his or her story.
2. Clear your mind.
3. Know when to use open and closed questions.
4. Demonstrate your understanding of their story.
5. Watch your language.
6. Embrace feelings.

# Let Patients Tell Their Story

Physicians' concerns about their lack of time is one of the biggest barriers to effective listening. They worry that if patients are allowed to talk, they will never stop. This worry is unfounded. In a study of 335 doctor-patient interactions, Langewitz et al (9) found that, when not interrupted, the average amount of time patients spent presenting their initial concern to an internist was 92 seconds. The same study found that 78% of the patients finished talking in two minutes, and only 2% of patients talked for more than five minutes. Another study found that when patients were allowed to speak uninterrupted, on average they spoke for a total of 32 seconds (10). The longest any patient spoke in this study was two minutes. The moral of this story is to let your patients do the talking. The overwhelming majority will self-regulate in a time-efficient manner.

## *Suggested Rule of Thumb: Be Prepared to Let Your Patient Speak Uninterrupted for Three Minutes*

Having a realistic time-frame in mind going into an exam room will help provide a structure for the interaction, help you feel a sense of control, and invite collaboration between you and your patient. A reasonable rule of thumb is to allow your patient to speak uninterrupted for up to three minutes. Your patient will feel like you have listened to them, and you will learn more of what you need to know to help them address their concerns. But how do you listen?

## *Clear Your Mind and Close Your Mouth*

Clearing your mind and closing your mouth will help you start to be a better listener. But once a person starts talking, how do you keep listening? We have all had the experience of trying to listen to a patient and found that instead we were thinking about something altogether different such as another patient or one of our children. It is normal for your mind to wander. The key is to lasso it and return your attention to the person in front of you once you notice it drifting away.

Listening is not a spectator sport. True listening requires that you be engaged in what your patient is telling you. This has been termed "active listening" or "empathic listening." Two of the goals of listening are to help your patient feel understood and to get the information you need to help your patient. But how do you do it? In addition to clearing your mind and closing your mouth, it is important to be strategic in how and when you do speak.

## *Open or Closed? The Question Is Yours*

Most first-year medical students learn the difference between open-ended and closed-ended questions. Open-ended questions are general and aim to elicit

Table **4-1**

# Open-Ended vs. Closed-Ended Questions

| Open-Ended Questions | Closed-Ended Questions |
|---|---|
| **1.** How can I be helpful to you? | **1.** What day did you first start feeling ill? |
| **2.** What else is concerning you? | **2.** Where exactly is the pain? |
| **3.** What factors do you think might be making your pain worse? Or better? | **3.** What medicines are you taking? |

more than one-word responses, giving your patient the choice on how much to disclose. Closed-ended questions elicit short responses. The purpose of closed ended-questions is to get a direct answer to your question. Examples of each type of question are listed in Table 4-1.

The type of question posed should match the type of response desired. Some suggest starting the interview with open-ended questions to build rapport and gather a wide range of information, and then proceed to more closed-ended questions to facilitate making the differential diagnosis (3). The following example illustrates how a physician moves from open-ended to closed-ended questions while interviewing a patient in order to make a diagnosis.

> MD: *Good morning Mrs. Kramer. What brings you in today?* (open-ended question)
>
> P: *Well, I have been having difficulty sleeping.*
>
> MD: *What do you think has been making it difficult for you to sleep?* (open-ended question)
>
> P: *I wake up many times during the night, usually to go to the bathroom.*
>
> MD: *Hmm, how long has this been going on?* (closed-ended question—starts thinking about a diagnosis, but does not want to jump to conclusions)
>
> P: *At least one month.*
>
> MD: *Are you having any other health problems?* (open-ended question to keep the differential diagnosis broad)
>
> P: *Yes, actually, I find that I am very thirsty. Also, I have some periods of light-headedness.*
>
> MD: *This is quite helpful. In your family, does anyone have diabetes?* (closed-ended question intended to hone in on a diagnosis.)

The skillful use of both open-ended and closed-ended questions can help you accomplish the goals of building a good relationship with your patient and obtain the information you need. Once you obtain needed information, the next step is to ensure understanding.

## Do I Understand?

Asking the right question is an important start, but you also need to show that you understand the response. This will accomplish at least two goals. First, it will clarify whether you really do understand what you have been told. Second, it will demonstrate that you are interested in what your patient is saying, that you have been listening, and that you are open to corrective feedback. Summarizing what you have heard and repeating it in terms your patient can understand will accomplish these goals. "So, Mrs. Robbins, it sounds like you have cold symptoms that have progressed into a nasty cough" will get you further than "This appears to be some variant of a rhinovirus with possible bronchitis."

## Watch Your Language

Medical jargon impairs patients' understanding of what you are saying. A lack of understanding, combined with patients' reluctance to admit confusion (11), is a breeding ground for a poor relationship. While it can be difficult to transition from the typical daily discourse that relies on medical terminology with colleagues to using plain language with patients, it is worthwhile. Patients want to know and understand what is going on with their bodies (12). Speaking to patients in a language they can understand will help you build a stronger working relationship. When it is necessary to use medical language, such as when providing a diagnosis, consider writing it down so the patient will not have to struggle with trying to remember an unfamiliar term.

## Feelings

The expression of feelings in clinical encounters can be complicated (13). While we all welcome our patients expressing positive emotions like happiness or gratitude, it can be uncomfortable for a physician if a patient expresses intense sadness or anger. You may have feelings of your own in response to what is happening with your patient. Should you cry? Laugh? Show anger? There are no clear guidelines for working with intense feelings in patient encounters. Using the ARCH principles (Acceptance, Respect, Curiosity, Honesty), which we presented in Chapter 3, can be helpful in guiding you to respond to intense emotion.

Acceptance of your patient's emotions, even when you find them inappropriate or disturbing, will help you listen to your patient. It is not your job to take away negative emotions. Patients are responsible for their feelings just as you are responsible for yours.

Respect can be demonstrated by accepting patients as they are. Imagine having a patient sobbing in your office in response to bad news you just delivered, thinking "This is uncomfortable, how can I get her to stop?" versus "She will be alright. Crying is part of being sad." Allowing her to continue to cry is respectful and will let her know that you can tolerate her feelings, even if you do not fully understand them.

Sometimes it is difficult to know what your patient is feeling. Acting in a curious manner by asking questions can be helpful. Labeling a feeling in a curious way ("I wonder if you might be feeling anxious?") will let your patient know that you are interested in her feelings and provide a chance to clarify her experience. "No, I am not anxious, I am just really sad that this disease has come back."

Honesty in the context of a professional relationship can help strengthen your relationship with your patient. "I am sorry your disease has come back" is an empathic and honest response to your patient. Physicians worry about expressing too much emotion but we are not aware of any reliable "emotionometer" to tell you when enough is enough. While there are inappropriate extremes for physicians in the expression of emotion, the grey zone in between these extremes is where most people operate.

# The Sounds of Silence

Silence in clinical encounters can be difficult to tolerate. We consistently hear from clinicians that silence drives them crazy. The reason silence is so difficult to tolerate is because of the uncertainty. When a patient is silent you do not know what he or she is thinking or feeling. An example from one of our early training experiences will help to illustrate this point.

During the first year of doctoral training, one of us was doing a clinical rotation on a spinal cord injury unit of a major metropolitan hospital and was assigned a newly arrived 28-year-old man who had been involved in a motor vehicle accident that resulted in complete quadriplegia. The patient, Bill, had a long history of drug and alcohol abuse and was intoxicated at the time of his injury. He was disruptive on the unit and he was loud, used foul language, and frequently made inappropriate, sexual comments to the nurses.

In the first session the rookie therapist wheeled Bill down the hall to a private consultation room. When they got settled, the therapist asked a few simple questions and Bill looked out the window in silence. After 50 grueling minutes of this, the therapist finally wheeled Bill back to his room. Bill had not spoken a word during the entire session.

Later that day the therapist-in-training met with his clinical supervisor and recounted the sweat-filled session. The supervisor looked at him and said,

*"You are not listening to him."*

*"Listening to him? Apparently you aren't listening to me. He didn't say anything! There was nothing to listen to!"* was the incredulous reply.

*"Your patient's silence made you so anxious that you tried to soothe your own anxiety by firing questions at him. The more questions you fired, the more he withdrew. The next time you meet with him, try to listen to what he is telling you."*

Two sessions later Bill finally broke the silence by looking out the window and saying:

*"It sure is a nice day."*

So what was Bill "saying?" He was saying that he needed to be in control. As soon as his neophyte therapist recognized that, they built a productive and collaborative relationship.

But what about a situation in which you have limited time and your patient is silent? It is acceptable for a physician to set limits around the silence. After a few minutes (remember, most patients express what they have to say in less than three minutes) it is appropriate to give your patient feedback on what you have been hearing. You can break the silence in a curious and respectful way by saying something like:

*"At a time like this, it can be hard to know what to say. I was wondering what you are thinking (or feeling)?"* or, *"This is difficult to talk about. I wonder if you need some time before we can continue to talk about this?"*

Sometimes patients will tell you what they are experiencing; other times they need privacy and will say nothing. If a patient chooses privacy, then you can move the encounter along by saying"

*"Is there anything else I can do to help you today?"*

If the answer is no, then suggest a reasonable timeframe for follow-up. Staying connected to a patient, even when you may not fully understand them, is a key part of listening well.

## Staying Connected

Staying connected to your patients involves understanding their view of the ongoing problems and agreeing on a way to proceed. This may involve scheduling follow-up office visits, telephone or email contact, or unscheduled visits when the patient deems them necessary. It may also include contacts with other professionals in your office including nurses, nurse practitioners, or other health professionals. The point of staying connected is to let your patients know that you will not abandon them and that you are invested in their ongoing care. This is an essential component to developing a trusting relationship with a patient.

## *Scenario #2 Revisited*

In Scenario #2, the physician did a good job of starting the interview in a respectful manner. The physician was surprised by the outburst of tears after he asked the patient how she was. Now, let us follow the interaction to see how to apply the elements of listening.

After Mrs. Robbins burst into tears, her physician tried to use a little humor ("Is it my tie?") to soothe his patient and himself. The patient, Mrs. Robbins, laughed through her tears and responded,

> *"No. I am so embarrassed. I'm sorry."*
>
> **Her physician responds:** *"No need to apologize. I am glad you feel comfortable to express yourself. What brings you in today?"* (Open-ended question)
>
> *"I have this terrible cold and I was wondering if there is anything you can do to help me get rid of this?"*
>
> *"Can you tell me how long you have been feeling like this?"* (closed-ended question)
>
> *"About one week. It started with a tightness in my chest. The next morning, I think that was last Tuesday, I woke up and just felt terrible. My nose was running and I had a terrible headache. I usually don't get this sick. The kids have been sick over the past few weeks but now I guess it's my turn. So, anyway, I had a runny nose and headache and then I developed a cough on Saturday. I am coughing all the time."*
>
> *"Have you had any fevers?"* (closed-ended question)
>
> *"No."*
>
> *"When you cough, is it productive? Do you bring up any phlegm?"* (closed-ended questions)
>
> *"A little; it's yellow."*
>
> *"So, you have had a cold with a runny nose for about one week and a cough that produces yellow phlegm for about three days* (demonstrates understanding). *Is there anything else you think I should know?"* (open-ended question)
>
> *"Well,* (pauses—MD refrains from speaking to give Mrs. Robbins a chance to talk). *No, nothing else."*

The physician senses that Mrs. Robbins has more to say and responds,

> *"It seems like there might be something else you want to tell me"* (encourages patient to tell her story).

> *"I have been pretty stressed lately. My friends tell me the reason I got this cold is because of the stress."*

> *"What is causing your stress?"*

> *"It's nothing, actually."*

The physician continues to sense that there is more to her story and tries to facilitate the conversation.

> *"I wonder, if it's nothing, then why did you cry when I first came in the room?"* (introduces feelings into the conversation)

Mrs. Robbins bursts into tears again.

> *"I am so embarrassed. It's just that my marriage is hitting a rough patch and I am worried about it. I haven't really talked to anyone about it and I don't know why I can't control myself in here."*

> *"Would you like to tell me more about it?"* (open-ended question encouraging patient to tell her story)"

> *"Well, I found out that my husband has been unfaithful. I can't believe it. We have been married for 10 years. I am trying to keep a happy face on around the house for the kids, but I feel like I am going to explode inside. I don't know why I am rambling on about it here, I really don't talk about it to anyone. At first I talked to some of my friends but they weren't very helpful."* (becomes silent)

The physician waits a few minutes and then says,

> *"It sounds like you don't know what to do."*

> *"Exactly. I have no idea what I'm supposed to do."*

> *"Do you have any thoughts on how I might be helpful to you?"* (open-ended question intended to facilitate the conversation)

> *"I have been thinking about counseling. I think I need to talk to someone who can help me straighten out my head. Do you know any good counselors?"*

> *"I do know some very good therapists and I will write down their names and phone numbers before you leave. As for your cold, rest, fluids, and over-the-counter cold medicines should help to get you through. Is there anything else I can do for you today?"*

*"No, thanks."*

*"I think we should schedule a follow-up visit for a few weeks just to see how you are doing. What do you think?"*

*"That would be helpful. Thanks again."*

This physician has effectively built a relationship with Mrs. Robbins by being respectful and by listening well. He let her tell her story and then demonstrated his understanding of the problem. He accepted Mrs. Robbins feelings even though they were confusing at the start of the interview. By being patient and inquisitive, he was able to elicit the entire story.

**Summary**

As effective as the basic tools we just presented can be, there are still situations where impasses between doctors and patients can emerge. In the discussions we had with doctors as part of preparing this book, as well as from our collective clinical experiences, we have identified six types of cases that are particularly troubling to practicing physicians. These cases include: the patient who wants a medical intervention to solve lifestyle-induced health problems, the angry patient, patients with unexplained symptoms who insist that the doctor do something, emotionally volatile family members, ethical dilemmas that mask underlying communication problems, and, finally, patients whose medical complaints are driven by psychological factors. Next, we will show you how to use the basics we just presented along with our models to see, understand, and resolve these difficult cases.

In this chapter we have:

- Presented the basics for building a trusting relationship with your patient
- Outlined effective components of listening
- Stressed the importance of staying connected to your patients
- Showed how to use all of the above to avoid an impasse with your patients

# References

1. **Minuchin S.** Families and Family Therapy. Cambridge, MA: Harvard University Press; 1974.

2. **Cohen-Cole SA, Bird J.** The Medical Interview: The Three-Function Approach, 2nd ed. Philadelphia; Mosby: 2000.

3. **Silverman J, Kurtz S, Draper J.** Skills for Communicating with Patients. San Francisco: Radcliffe Publishing; 2005.

4. **McDaniel SH, Campbell TL, Hepworth J, Lorenz A.** Family Oriented Primary Care, 2nd ed. New York: Springer; 2005.

5. **Buckman, R.** How to Break Bad News. Baltimore: Johns Hopkins University Press; 1992.

6. **Beckman HB, Frankel RM.** The effect of physician behavior on the collection of data. Ann Intern Med. 1984;101:692-6.

7. **Starfield B, Wray C, Hess K, et al.** The influence of patient-practitioner agreement on outcome of care. Am J Public Health. 1981;71:127-31.

8. **Stewart M, Donner A, McWHinney IR, et al.** The impact of patient-centered care on patient outcomes in family practice. Thames Valley Family Practice Research Unit, Ontario; 1997.

9. **Langewitz W, Denz M, Keller A, et al.** Spontaneous talking time at start of consultation in outpatient clinic. Cohort study. BMJ. 2002;325:682-3.

10. **Marvel MK, Epstein RM, Flowers K, Beckman HB.** Soliciting the patient's agenda: have we improved? JAMA. 1999;281:283-7.

11. **Svarstad BL.** The Doctor-Patient Encounter: An Observational Study of Communication and Outcome. Madison: University of Wisconsin Press; 1974.

12. **Faden R, Becker C, Lewis C, et al.** Disclosure of information to patients in medical care. Med Care. 1981;19:718-33.

13. **Halpern, J.** Empathy and Patient-Physician Conflicts. J Gen Intern Med. 2007;22:696-700.

# Part III
# Responding to Difficult Relationships

# Chapter 5
# When All You Know Isn't Enough: Dealing with Chronic Illness

## "Doctor, Can't You Just Give Me Something?"

Tom White is not a medical success story. No matter how many times he has spoken to his doctor, his health problems persist. As a young man, Tom was active and physically fit. He worked in manual labor jobs and played basketball every week with childhood friends. His competitive spirit motivated him to jog and ride his bicycle to stay "game ready." At the age of 30, Tom landed his first telephone customer service job. Tom's friends would often comment that he could talk to a wall and this talent helped him succeed in a

### Key Terms
- Know your role
- Breaking the cycle

job that many would consider boring. Tom loved to talk to customers on the phone and use his problem-solving skills to help resolve their concerns. Tom also enjoyed going out for a few cold ones after work with his buddies. Gradually, Tom stopped playing basketball and exercising. He got married and had two children, which further limited his time to exercise. As Tom progressed through his 30s, so too did his waist size.

Tom's medical problems began at age 40 when he developed low back pain after his weight increased from 180 to 215 pounds. He sat all day long at work, and his exercise became limited to playing with his children and doing home repairs. His diet was what some would consider "all American"—high fat, low fruits and vegetables. His blood pressure also started to creep up. By age 45 Tom weighed 240 pounds and he was diagnosed with Type II diabetes. He began to complain of pain in his knees. After tolerating these various discomforts for some time, Tom went to his internist and said he felt like he was "falling apart."

Tom's internist, Peter Davis, was a self-made man. He was the son of immigrant parents who worked multiple low-skilled jobs to support their two sons and provide opportunities they could only dream of. Peter learned the value of commitment and hard work early in his life when he worked any job he could find. He mowed lawns, shoveled snow, delivered newspapers, painted fences, and anything else that would generate income. He also excelled in the classroom and he was accepted into an ivy-league undergraduate program in biology. His academic success continued as he completed medical school and residency training. He proudly displayed his diplomas in his office, but he carried himself in a quiet, dignified way. His demeanor resembled his sport coats; tightly woven tweed that was warm and comfortable. His patients liked him and were consistently impressed with his quick mind. But Peter Davis had little tolerance for patients who did not do their part in maintaining their health, and Tom White fell into this category.

When Dr. Davis last saw Tom White he conducted a complete physical exam and ordered x-rays of Tom's low back and both knees and an MRI of his lumbar spine. All radiographic findings were normal, except for some mild degenerative changes in each knee. Mr. White begins his current office visit by voicing frustration to Dr. Davis about his health.

> *"I'm really getting sick and tired of feeling so lousy all the time. I enjoy my family and my job, but between all the work of this diabetes thing, and the pain in my back and knees, I feel like an old jalopy. I need help."*

> **Dr. Davis replies,** *"Well Tom, you do have a number of health concerns and I will do all I can to help you. But one question we also need to ask is what you can do for yourself?"*

> *"I think I do quite a bit for myself. I check my blood sugars all the time and give myself insulin injections. I also try to watch my diet, but a guy's got to eat! What else am I supposed to do?"*

*"As we've talked about before, losing weight would cer-
tainly help your health in many different ways."*

*"Now you sound like my wife! Look, I'm doing my best. I was
hoping you might have something else to help me."*

*"Like what?"*

*"Diet pills or something like that."*

# Physician-as-Expert

Mr. White views Dr. Davis as the expert and wants him to solve his health
problems. Dr. Davis is willing to accept the role of expert, but believes that
Tom must be an active participant in the process. As Tom continues to look
to his physician to fix him, Dr. Davis starts to feel powerless. Figure 5-1 uses
the Physician-as-Expert Model to illustrate this interaction.

In response to Mr. White's request for diet pills, Dr. Davis tries to set a
limit.

*"Tom, I typically don't prescribe diet pills for overweight pa-
tients. There are many more healthy ways to lose weight."*

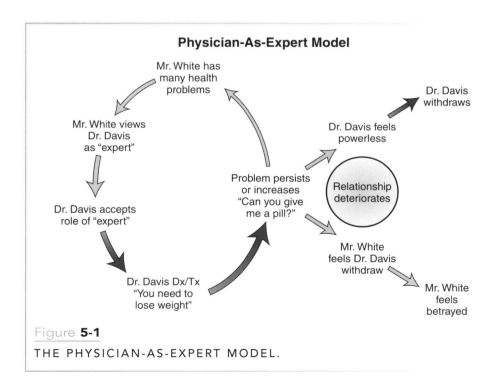

**Physician-As-Expert Model**

Mr. White has many health problems

Mr. White views Dr. Davis as "expert"

Dr. Davis accepts role of "expert"

Dr. Davis Dx/Tx "You need to lose weight"

Problem persists or increases "Can you give me a pill?"

Relationship deteriorates

Dr. Davis feels powerless

Dr. Davis withdraws

Mr. White feels Dr. Davis withdraw

Mr. White feels betrayed

Figure **5-1**

THE PHYSICIAN-AS-EXPERT MODEL.

**Mr. White states his case.** *"Oh sure, exercise more and eat less. I know that. But it is really hard to get any exercise given my job and the demands of my family. If that actually worked, I wouldn't be here today."*

*"Tell me what type of exercise program you have tried."*

**Mr. White throws his arms up and says,** *"I'm not going to put out a lot of cash to one of those fancy gyms, if that's what you mean by an exercise program. Those guys just rip you off."*

*"Joining a gym is only one way of developing an exercise program. Other ways include…"*

*"I used to exercise all the time but how can I do that with this bum back and creaky knees? I mean, let's get real here."*

*"I think exercise will actually help your back and knees."*

*"How?"*

# Step 1: Seeing the Impasse

Dr. Davis' frustration escalates as he realizes that Mr. White is focused on having the doctor fix his problems. His frustration is a potential landmine if it leads Dr. Davis to take a rigid position toward Mr. White ("You must lose weight!"). This is the point where seeing the emerging impasse can help Dr. Davis to begin the transition from the Physician-as-Expert Model to the Physician-as-Collaborator Model. Dr. Davis finds this transition challenging because as he tries to educate Mr. White in ways to improve his health, he feels like his suggestions are being dismissed. Dr. Davis' initial response is to try harder to educate Mr. White about the benefits of weight loss.

*"Okay, let's look at your health problems and then consider options to help you feel better. You have Type II diabetes, borderline hypertension, back pain, and knee pain. You are also about 60 pounds overweight. Anything else?"*

*"I think you covered it all."*

*"When I look at each of these problems individually, and when I look at your overall health, there is one common thread running through it all."*

*"Good—now we are getting somewhere."*

*"Not so fast. The common thread I see is excess weight."*

*"You have been talking to my wife! I knew it!"*

*"No, I have not spoken to your wife. But if I did, it sounds like we would get along just fine. Seriously, Tom, your weight is the single biggest factor in both your short-term and long-term health."*

*"I know, I know. I have tried so many things and it just seems like I end up in the same place—fat and sore."*

**Davis tries to transition into a collaborative mode.** *"Tom, I think the question is—are you ready to change your lifestyle?"*

*"I have given that a lot of thought. I've even thought about getting one of those bypass operations. Not the one for your heart, the one for your stomach. What do you know about those operations?"*

*"You are not a candidate for gastric bypass surgery!"*

Dr. Davis thought he was making progress and felt deflated when Mr. White suggested gastric bypass surgery. Over the years, he has learned that one of his own internal warning signs of an impasse is feeling anger toward a patient. He sees that despite his efforts to educate Mr. White on the health benefits of weight loss, Mr. White continues to focus on medical solutions. Remaining in the Physician-as-Expert mode has left Dr. Davis feeling powerless because he sees the obvious route to health (lose weight), but Mr. White dismisses his recommendation. As Dr. Davis continues using the same approach, an impasse begins to emerge. Dr. Davis wants to build a collaborative relationship with Mr. White by including him in the process of improving his health but feels like the harder he tries, the more rigid Mr. White becomes. In order to transition from the Physician-as-Expert Model to the Physician-as-Collaborator Model, Dr. Davis must first understand why he is stuck.

# Step 2: Understanding the Impasse

We can use the Symptomatic Cycle framework to try to understand Dr. Davis' impasse with Mr. White. Figure 5-2 frames the interaction in the Symptomatic Cycle.

The Symptomatic Cycle illustrates how the doctor and patient are stuck on parallel and linear paths that lead to the same outcome. Unfortunately, all of their efforts are going toward problem solving rather than on building their relationship.

As the impasse emerges, both parties become more entrenched in their positions. The more Dr. Davis tries to help Tom, the more trapped and frustrated he feels by Tom's "stubborn" refusal to change his mind. Applying the universal principles can be a good starting point to diffuse the impasse and move the interaction in a collaborative direction (Box 5-1).

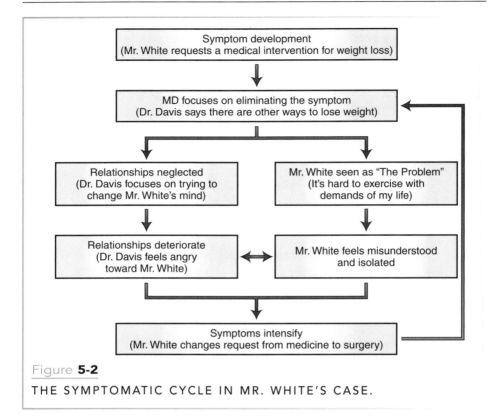

Figure **5-2**

THE SYMPTOMATIC CYCLE IN MR. WHITE'S CASE.

---

Box **5-1**

## Step 3: Responding to the Impasse

1. **Apply the Universal Principles**
   Know your Role
   Competence and Collaboration
2. **Use the ARCH**

---

# Applying the Universal Principles

## *Know Your Role*

Dr. Davis is experiencing a common situation that leads to frustration because he is unclear about his role with Mr. White. There is a subtle, but significant, struggle for control in the interactions between Mr. White and Dr. Davis. Each is asking the other to give something they are unwilling to provide. Dr. Davis is not going to prescribe diet pills or recommend surgery, and Mr. White is not going to start exercising. This leaves Dr. Davis not knowing how to help him. He feels powerless and may even feel that he is wasting his time with Mr. White. A key task for Dr. Davis then is to become aware of his role, limits, and function. He currently sees his role as one of providing solid advice to Mr. White on how to lose weight and trying to get Mr. White to change his approach to his health. Yet, despite his efforts, Mr. White continues to ignore his recommendations. One physician that we interviewed for this book spoke about how he deals with patients who ignore what he has to say:

> *"It used to really irk me when I made a recommendation and somebody didn't follow it. But now I think my role with patients has changed. I am not responsible for that patient doing what I recommend. Before, if I recommended that a person stop smoking or that they exercise or lose weight or take this pill, and they didn't do it, I used to take that personally. And three months later when the patient's blood pressure wasn't what it should be, I would think 'That patient's going to have a stroke, and it will be my fault if I don't help save him.' Over the years I've become much more of an advisor. I think I'm better at helping people understand the rationale for doing something and I am a more effective physician. Patients still often decide that they don't want to take my advice, but it almost never bothers me.*
>
> *"I think part of this equation is that people who go into medicine have a strong sense of responsibility. I do think, deep down, we feel responsible for everything good and bad that happens to our patients."*

This physician describes his progression from feeling completely responsible for the patient's health to more clearly defining his role as an advisor to the patient. He still acts as an expert, but no longer believes that he must take responsibility for the outcome. By clarifying his role (advisor), limits (the patient decides), and function ("I'm better at helping people understand the rationale for doing something"), he has decreased his frustration in dealing with patients. But how does a physician do this with a patient like Tom, who is so rigidly attached to the idea of a medical intervention to help him lose weight? The answer lies in using the universal principles to develop a strategic approach to building a collaborative relationship with Mr. White.

## Breaking the Cycle: Competence and Collaboration

Dr. Davis' first step in trying to resolve the impasse is to develop a clear framework for how to approach Mr. White. If Dr. Davis feels responsible for Mr.

White losing weight, they are in for a long and frustrating relationship. If he views himself as an expert who can provide Mr. White with accurate information, support, and encouragement, he will be in a better position to help him.

Highlighting competencies is a good way to approach anyone when an impasse is developing. This can be done by incorporating the ARCH (acceptance, respect, curiosity, and honesty) into the conversation.

Returning to the outpatient visit, Dr. Davis collects his thoughts and tries to apply the ARCH.

> "Tom I know you just want to feel better, and I also know you have tried to improve your health (acceptance and respect). I have always been impressed with your problem-solving abilities (highlight competencies). When you talk about your job, one of the things you say you like the most is solving problems. What puzzles me though (curiosity), is that when it comes to your health, you seem to be focused only on medical solutions."

> "You mean with the pills and the operation?"

> "Exactly."

> "Well, I have heard from other people that those things can be really helpful."

Dr. Davis senses a shift in the conversation and decides to take a risk by being open and honest.

> "In certain people they can be helpful. But for you, we are so focused on medical interventions, we are not considering other things that can be a lot safer and more gratifying for you. Quite frankly, I really want to help you but I feel like I am working against you on this. Since I have told you that I won't give you diet pills or recommend surgery, I am unsure what I can do for you."

In this exchange, Dr. Davis has stated the problem directly in an effort to shift the discussion to a collaborative mode and clarify his role. Figure 5-3 uses the Physician-as-Collaborator model to illustrate the shift.

Dr. Davis' task is to move away from the Physician-as-Expert Model and into the Physician-as-Collaborator Model. As Dr. Davis focuses on being collaborative, and not controlling ("Why won't you just do as I recommend?"), the tone of the conversation changes.

Mr. White continues:

> "If you won't give me diet pills and you don't think I should get bypass surgery, I really don't know how you can help me."

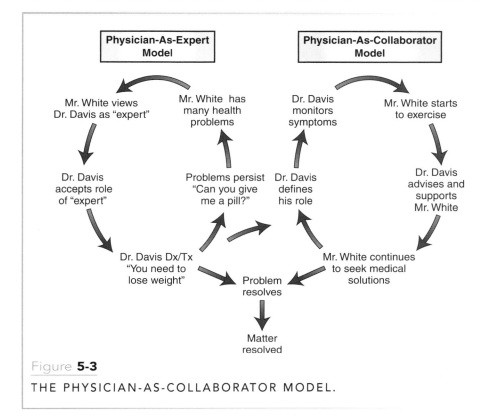

Figure **5-3**

THE PHYSICIAN-AS-COLLABORATOR MODEL.

Trying to stay in a collaborative mode, Dr. Davis responds:

> *"It would be worth giving that some thought. How about if you return in a month and we can talk more about how I can help you."*

One month passes and Mr. White returns.

> *"Well doctor Davis, I haven't lost any weight."*

Feeling a pang of defeat, Dr. Davis tries to remain collaborative.

> *"Have you thought about our conversation since we last met?"*
>
> *"Not really."*

Puzzled, Dr. Davis reminds him about their last conversation.

> *"We were talking about how I might help you."*
>
> *"Oh yeah, right. Hmmm, I really don't know."*
>
> *"Can I make some suggestions?"*
>
> *"Sure."*

Dr. Davis uses this opportunity to be clear about his role, limits, and function.

> *"I have given a good bit of thought to how I could help you. My job is to help you to get healthy and stay healthy. My job is also to protect you from potential harm, if possible. I think I have been clear that losing weight is the first step to returning you to a more healthy state. I don't see medicine or surgery as being the best way to get you there. That said, I think the best way I can help you is to continue to offer my advice on ways to improve your health (clarifies role). It is up to you to decide what to do with my advice."*
>
> *"So, basically, the ball is in my court?"*

Dr. Davis then tries to build a bridge from Tom's competencies in life to his medical problems.

> *"Tom, you were a good basketball player in your day. If you were teaching someone how to shoot a foul shot, how would you do it?"*
>
> *"What does this have to do with my health?"*
>
> *"Bear with me—how would you teach someone to shoot a foul shot?"*
>
> *"First, I would explain how to get their legs set in the proper position. Then I would tell them how to focus their attention on the rim. Then I would show them how to hold the ball and release it in a smooth motion."*
>
> *"And that would be enough to make someone a good foul-throw shooter?"*
>
> *"Well, no, of course not. They would have to go out and practice!"*
>
> *"Right. I can tell you everything I know, but at the end of the day, you have to go out and practice. I can be your coach, but you have to play the game."*
>
> *"I get it. That makes sense."*

Dr. Davis stays in his role as a coach to Mr. White.

> *"I have some suggestions for an exercise plan that might be of help. I also have the name of a nutritionist who some of my patients have found helpful."*
>
> *"Okay, I'll take the information."*

While Mr. White agrees to take the information, he does not commit to change. Despite Mr. White being non-committal, Dr. Davis has successfully moved from conflict to collaboration. By defining his role, Dr. Davis has freed himself of the chess match of Mr. White trying to get a medical intervention and Dr. Davis trying to get him to change.

# Scenario Resolution

Mr. White started to walk in the mornings before work. He was unable to sustain the effort and stopped after a few weeks. He never contacted the nutritionist. Dr. Davis continues to see him and maintains a collaborative approach to caring for him by being clear about his role, limits, and function. He has grown to like Mr. White and remains hopeful that, at some point, he will initiate a committed effort to change his lifestyle. If that time arrives, Dr. Davis will be ready to help.

# Practice Points

The case of Tom White illustrates how to apply our models when a patient's lifestyle choices contribute to their health problems. Some more general lessons learned from this scenario that can be applied to other cases include:

1. **Know your own warning signs of being caught in an impasse.** Do you feel anger toward a patient, as did Dr. Davis? Do you find yourself not returning phone calls promptly? Are you withdrawing from your patient in other ways? The earlier you recognize your own signals, the sooner you will be able to make important adjustments to stay engaged with, as opposed to turning away from, your patient.

2. **Push for change, but focus on controlling your behavior, not your patient's.** It is possible to push for change without being seen as controlling by your patient. Being prepared for the possibility of multiple outcomes will help you to create a relationship that promotes change yet can tolerate the frustration of a lack of change.

3. **Know your role and limits.** By defining your role, you help your patient to clarify what they expect from you. By setting limits, you avoid the trap of trying to meet a need that you are unable to satisfy (Box 5-2).

Box **5-2**

# Internet Mania

One of the outgrowths of the Internet is that some patients arrive at their doctor's office armed with reams of information about a particular medical condition. While this can be helpful in many ways—it encourages patient involvement in their care, and it can be educational for patients and, at times, doctors—it also presents challenges for physicians. One challenge is that it can take a considerable amount of time to sift through the information and try to determine what is, and is not, credible. Another challenge is that a physician may feel like the patient is pitting the doctor's knowledge against the Internet information. As a result, remaining in a collaborative mode can be difficult. Here are some suggestions for working with these patients.

1. **Focus on Relationships:** Think about how the Internet information impacts your relationship with your patient, rather than being focused on the content of the information. Bringing the information to the visit is your patient's attempt to contribute to their getting well.

2. **Highlight Competencies:** Acknowledge to the patient how you admire their interest and curiosity in their own health. This demonstrates your interest in the patient and that you want to understand them.

3. **Be Curious:** If the Internet information is creating conflict between you and a patient (for example, by contradicting your recommendations) ask your patient, "How does this difference between your information and my recommendation affect you and impact us? For example, do you think there is something missing from my recommendations? Are you worried that I may be missing something? Are we at a point where we should seek input from another physician?"

4. **Remain collaborative:** The most important thing is to stay emotionally connected to your patient, not allowing disagreements to promote emotional withdrawal. Trust that your relationship can weather the storm of disagreement. Some physicians, in an attempt to be collaborative, provide lists of disease-specific websites to patients who prefer to get information from the Internet.

# Chapter **6**
# "You Are Not Helping Me!"

## Dealing with the Angry Patient

Julie Hennessy could best be described as a loner. At 36, she lives with her older brother and younger sister in the house in which they grew up. She has no real friends and has never had a romantic relationship. She is quiet and tends to keep to herself. With the exception of an occasional cold, she has enjoyed good health her entire life. That is about to change.

For the past five years Julie has been employed as an administrative assistant at a large corporation. One day at work she tried to lift a small box and felt intense pain in her low back and down her left leg. Several days later Julie went to her primary

> **Key Terms**
> - Isolation and disconnection
> - Focus on relationships

care physician, Dr. Cindy Russell, because the pain was not improving. Dr. Russell knew little about her but remembered her as a shy, pleasant person.

When Dr. Russell entered the exam room, she found Julie sitting in an awkward position, leaning toward the right side of her chair, and she appeared to have been crying. She re-introduced herself and asked Julie what had happened. Julie replied:

> "Well, I was at work and I bent over to pick up a box of papers to begin filing them. As soon as I started to straighten up, I heard this loud pop in my back and I felt this shooting pain down my left leg. It knocked me to the ground. I yelled and the other people around me gave me a look like 'What's wrong with you?' I kept my composure, but the pain was terrible. After an hour I told my supervisor because it wasn't getting any better. I also thought, you know how big companies can be, if I didn't tell them and I needed medical attention, they would just tell me I was lying. My supervisor told me to fill out some forms and if I needed to, I could go home to rest. That was two days ago and the pain is getting worse. I am really worried that something bad happened to my back."

After a thorough exam, Dr. Russell decided that conservative treatment was appropriate. She recommended physical therapy (PT) and a return visit in two weeks. She also prescribed anti-inflammatory medication and an oral narcotic for pain control.

## The Pain Continues

Five days later Dr. Russell received a call from Julie stating that she went to physical therapy and that it made her much worse and she would not go back. Dr. Russell then ordered plain radiographic films and an MRI of Julie's lumbar spine. The plain films were normal, but the MRI showed a disc herniation at L5-S1. Dr. Russell then referred Julie to a spine surgeon for an evaluation. The spine surgeon decided that a discectomy was an appropriate intervention, and the surgery was performed. Julie reported considerable pain relief for a period of six months, but her pain gradually returned, at which point her spine surgeon recommended PT. She went to PT but got no relief. After four PT sessions Julie reported increasing pain and stated that she would not return for more therapy. The spine surgeon ordered more radiographic studies in an attempt to figure out the cause of her pain. Though the films were not conclusive, the spine surgeon believed that instability of the lumbar spine was the likely cause of the pain. He discussed the case with several colleagues and, though slightly reluctant, he decided that a spinal fusion was an appropriate surgery. The surgery was performed approximately 15 months after Julie's initial injury. The surgeon fused L-4, L-5, and L-5, S-1 using bone grafts from Julie's hip and from cadavers.

Post-operatively, Julie reported intense pain and refused to get out of bed. High doses of narcotics were administered, but her pain complaints continued. Julie reported that her left leg radiculopathy was worse post-operatively than at any time since she was injured. The spine surgeon recommended more PT, but Julie refused. Twelve weeks after the spinal fusion, the spine surgeon referred Julie to a pain clinic for help. He told her that he had nothing further to offer her and the pain clinic might be able to help her manage the pain. Julie's parting comment to the surgeon was,

> "Well, it must be nice to be able to just send your mistakes to other people."

# Next Stop, the Pain Clinic

Sue Torres decided to become a pain specialist during her anesthesia residency. She was drawn to the physiology and pharmacology of pain and felt compelled to specialize in pain management after witnessing so much unrelieved suffering during her training. However, about eight weeks into her pain fellowship, she feared that she had made a big mistake. Her vision was that her days would be filled relieving people's pain. Instead, what she found herself doing was renewing prescriptions and doing procedures, many of which did not work, on people who could not find any end to their suffering. She wondered where she would find the patience to work with such misery. Julie Hennessy was about to test her patience even further.

Ms. Hennessy arrived 15 minutes early for her first pain clinic appointment. When she checked in with the receptionist, she did not make eye contact and she spoke in a low voice. The receptionist welcomed her to the clinic and offered her a cup of coffee. Julie looked away and then sat in the corner of the waiting room, away from all of the other patients. When the receptionist gave the nurse Julie's paperwork, she commented, "She seems like a wounded animal."

When Dr. Torres entered Ms. Hennessy's room and introduced herself, Julie quickly spoke her mind.

> "That surgeon ruined me. All he wanted was the money. How does he expect me to live with pain like this? I need help and I hope you are smart enough to give it to me. I believe the problem is that the hardware that butcher put in my back is irritating my nerves and causing all of this pain. I've had just about enough of doctors. The doctors have ruined me and I may have to finish the job."

Dr. Torres did not know how to respond, but remained calm and stayed on task. She did a physical exam and explained that she believed that Julie had "failed back syndrome." She explained that medications could be helpful, but that it was important that Julie actively try to return to a functional life. Julie was quiet but appeared to be listening. When Dr. Torres asked Julie if she had any questions, she said no. Dr. Torres prescribed a long-acting narcotic and gabapentin for the neuropathic pain and Julie left the clinic without comment.

# "You're Not Helping Me"

One week later Julie called the clinic asking to speak with a physician. When the receptionist asked her the nature of the problem, Julie screamed,

*"You people are not helping me! I must be seen today!"*

The receptionist was flustered and added Julie onto the schedule without checking with the attending physician. When Dr. Torres found out about this addition onto an already full schedule, she felt her shoulders tense and her head started to throb. When Julie arrived for her clinic appointment later that morning, here is how her interaction went:

*"So, Julie, what seems to be the problem today?"*

*"You gave me these medicines and they are not helping my pain. I need something to control this pain. I told you the last time that the hardware in my back is the problem. Can you take it out?"*

*"Sometimes it takes time for certain medicines to be effective. I'm not surprised that you have not yet felt relief. As far as the hardware is concerned, I am not the physician who takes out hardware. If that is appropriate, a spine surgeon would be the one to perform that procedure."*

*"My last spine surgeon said the hardware was stable so it could not be the cause of my pain. And who do those people who answer your phones think they are, telling me I can't talk to a doctor? I'm the patient. I'm paying the bills here!"*

*"Now just a minute, the people who work in this clinic are very dedicated to helping everyone who comes here, including you. As far as I'm concerned you were out of line in the way you spoke to my staff earlier. I will not tolerate that behavior from anyone, including you."*

# Step 1: Seeing the Impasse

Julie's increasingly antagonistic behavior understandably angered Dr. Torres. While this is not surprising, it is important to see how Dr. Torres' anger toward Julie contributed to an impasse. The Physician-as-Expert Model in Figure 6-1 shows how their interactions have become derailed by conflict.

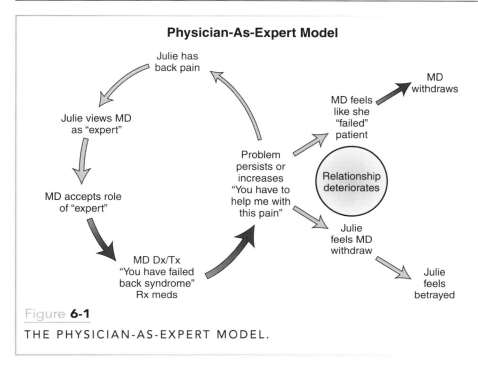

**Physician-As-Expert Model**

Figure **6-1**

THE PHYSICIAN-AS-EXPERT MODEL.

As the impasse emerges, the medical staff shifts their focus from Julie's pain to her irritating behavior. This behavior then distracts the medical staff from their primary role of providing pain relief. Once this pattern is identified, the next step in moving toward resolution is to understand what is sustaining the destructive cycle.

# Step 2: Understanding the Impasse

While Julie has only been to the clinic for a few visits, the efforts of the medical staff to help Ms. Hennessy have backfired. Despite approaching her with the best of intentions, she continues to be rude and disrespectful toward them. This has made it hard for the staff to reach out to her. As a result, the staff have become angry and started to withdraw from her. The Symptomatic Cycle illustrates how this pattern is sustained (Figure 6-2).

The cycle that is evolving is driven by Julie demanding pain relief and the medical staff focusing on her disruptive behavior. While the demands for pain relief escalate, the staff members withdraw because they feel increasingly angry toward her and powerless to help.

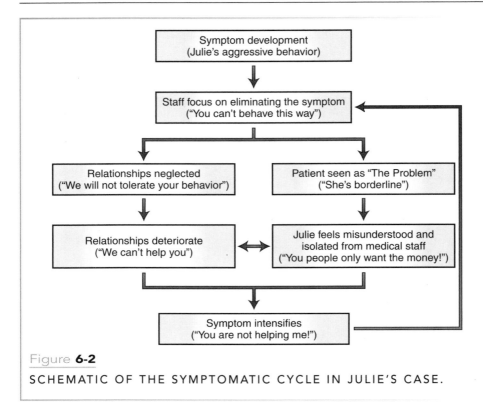

Figure **6-2**

SCHEMATIC OF THE SYMPTOMATIC CYCLE IN JULIE'S CASE.

# Enough Is Enough

Dr. Torres was struggling with intense anger toward Julie. After six months of trying to help her, she decided it was time to return Julie to the care of her primary care physician, Dr. Russell. This decision was driven by the sense that she had nothing to offer Julie and she was fed up with her tirades. Dr. Torres was unknowingly abandoning Julie. Fortunately, Dr. Torres decided to talk to Julie before discharging her from the clinic.

> *"Julie, we have been seeing you for six months in this clinic and we don't seem to have helped you much."*
>
> *"What are you saying?"*
>
> *"I am just not sure we can help you."*
>
> *"You have to help me! No one else will. How can I live like this?"*
>
> **Dr. Torres tries to remain calm.** *"I am not sure what else I can offer."*

> Crying now, Ms. Hennessy pleads for help. *"I know you are trying. But no one is listening to me. I have told you and every other doctor that the cause of my pain is the hardware in my back. Why won't anyone listen to me?"*

Dr. Torres is in a bind. She wants to have this problem go away but is troubled by a nagging sense of guilt. She is angry at Julie and feels powerless to help her, yet she does not know what to do next. Applying the universal principles can help provide a map to navigate this dilemma (Box 6-1).

# Isolation and Disconnection Exacerbate Psychological Distress

One of the obvious aspects of this scenario is that Ms. Hennesy is isolated and disconnected from people. Her behavior drives people away. While the office staff and nurses have tried to be kind and accommodating to her, there is clearly a wedge between them. The isolation and disconnection between Ms. Hennesy and the medical staff is what is driving the impasse.

As the impasse continues, Dr. Torres feels increasingly angry, and this isolates her from Ms. Hennesy. In addition to having to deal with her abrasiveness, the nursing and administrative staff are looking toward Dr. Torres to fix the problem. Several support staff have said to Dr. Torres that they believe Ms. Hennesy should be discharged from the clinic. While she agrees in part, she also feels an obligation to keep trying to help her patient. The problem for Dr. Torres is that she is not sure what to do next. Focusing on developing helpful relationships is a good place to start.

# Focus on Relationships

The key task when facing isolation and disconnection is to decrease one's own isolation by focusing on developing collaborative relationships. Dr. Torres decided to call Ms. Hennessy's primary care doctor and spine surgeon to talk with them about Julie's case. She did not know what she would get out of the conversations, but she saw no other options. After speaking to each of the physicians they all agreed that a team meeting might be helpful. The meeting consisted of Dr. Torres, the primary care physician Dr. Russell, the spine surgeon (SS), and several clinic nurses (N). Here is how the meeting went.

> **Dr. Torres:** *Thank you for coming to this meeting. I think the goal of this meeting is to discuss if there are ways we can help Julie.*
>
> **SS:** *Yeah, send her to psych.*
>
> **N:** *I agree. She's borderline, what do you expect?*
>
> **Dr. Russell:** *She calls my office and wants to be seen all the time. I don't know what to do.*
>
> **Dr. Torres:** *I don't either, but I can tell you that my staff has had enough of her. She is very abusive toward them. Before we send her to a psychiatrist, though, I think we need to make sure that medically we have done all we can.*
>
> **SS:** *I don't know how you put up with her. I'm convinced she is going to sue me one day.*

## *See Your Role in the Impasse*

Thus far in the meeting, the conversation has been directed toward Julie's troubling behavior. The risk in keeping the focus on the patient's behavior is that the physicians do not see how they may be inadvertently contributing to the impasse. As we pointed out in earlier chapters, in the face of feeling powerless, medical staff may blame the patient and make a psychiatric diagnosis. This is an attempt to alleviate the guilt associated with not being able to help Julie. It also cuts off the possibility of developing a collaborative relationship with her. In this case, Dr. Russell made a comment in the meeting that shifted the tone.

> **Dr. Russell:** *I agree with all of this psych stuff. She is a bit of a nut. But one thing that has always bugged me is that she is not a typical pain patient. What I mean is, when she comes to see me she has never once asked for more narcotics. People who are this disruptive usually want more meds. She's never done that.*
>
> **Dr. Torres:** *That's interesting, because she has never done that with me either. I never thought about that.*
>
> **N:** *I agree, she is not your typical patient. One thing we said after her last visit was that even though she can be a real pain in the neck, there is something about her that pulls at your heart.*
>
> **Dr. Russell:** *I think it's her loneliness. Let's face it, even before this pain, her life seemed pretty miserable.*

The tone of the conversation has shifted because the medical staff has stopped blaming Ms. Hennessy and are starting to look beyond her disruptive behavior. This accomplishes two main goals. First, it decreases the anger toward her and second, it decreases each physician's isolation with his or her struggle over how to help Julie. By talking openly about the complexities of the case, Dr. Torres feels relief ("I'm not the only one who feels this way."), and this decreases her own sense of isolation. The physician's blind spot (as discussed in Chapter 3) has been exposed ("She's borderline—what do you expect?") and the result is that the physicians become more introspective. The meeting continues.

> **Dr. Torres:** *The last time I saw her she said something at the end of our meeting that has stayed with me. She said no one is listening to her.*
>
> **Dr. Russell:** *Do you think she is right? Are we listening to her?*
>
> **Dr. Torres:** *She keeps saying that the pain is caused by her hardware.*
>
> **SS:** *I've looked at her films closely. Her fusion is stable and there doesn't appear to be any nerve root impingement.*
>
> **Dr. Russell:** *So, she is not a surgical candidate?*
>
> **SS:** *I don't know. This is a tough one. Some people report that they do get pain relief when the hardware is removed, but there is not a lot of empirical support for this. What makes this so hard is that given all of the psychiatric stuff, it is hard to know if it is wise to expose her to surgical risks. The outcome could be the same.*
>
> **Dr. Torres:** *So, what do we do?*
>
> **SS:** *I could remove the hardware. It's not a big procedure. To be honest, if she wasn't such a whack job, I probably would have taken it out a long time ago.*

The group agrees to proceed with the surgical intervention. Dr. Torres then meets with Julie to explain the shift.

> *"Julie, last week I met with your surgeon and primary care doctor. We talked for a long time about how we could help you. We all agreed that you are only trying to get better and we admire that. We have decided that going ahead and removing the hardware is a reasonable thing to do even though it may not help your pain. You can set up an appointment with your surgeon to get this scheduled if that is what you want to do."*

Crying, Ms. Hennessy expresses thanks to Dr. Torres.

# Scenario Resolution

Julie had the surgical procedure to remove the hardware from her back. Her post-operative course was rocky. Once again, she reported excruciating post-operative pain. For the first three days after surgery she could be heard screaming in pain at the end of the hospital hallway. She was discharged to a rehabilitation hospital after one week. Two weeks later she returned home. Her surgeon managed her medications for one month. She then returned to the pain clinic for medication management. At that point her pain was improving and her narcotic requirement was half the pre-operative dose. After two months, Julie returned to Dr. Russell who managed her medications.

Six months later Julie arrived in the pain clinic unannounced. She brought a cake she had baked, and asked to see Dr. Torres. She told Dr. Torres that the cake was a simple thank you for all of the help she had received. Julie told the clinic staff that she was attending school to get an associates degree in information technology. She eventually completed the training program and found a full-time job at a local financial institution. She sees Dr. Russell monthly for medication refills. While she continues to have back pain and intermittent radiculopathy, she reports that the pain is at least 70% improved since the surgery.

# Practice Points

Dealing with angry patients is a challenge for all clinicians. While Julie's case may be more extreme than most, there are some key ideas from this scenario that can be applied to other cases:

1. **Anger is a smokescreen.** Anger is a secondary emotion that is driven by deeper feelings (1). Feelings such as fear, hurt, and powerlessness are the most common emotions that trigger anger. Listening for, and directly addressing, the primary emotions will help diffuse the anger.

2. **Be open to your patient's perspective.** Tuning into the feelings beneath the anger will help you to short-circuit the fight-or-flight response to angry patients. This will help you to become more open and flexible, thereby enhancing your ability to hear what they are trying to tell you.

3. **Anger hides "diamonds in the rough."** As doctors, we see people at their best and at their worst. By developing collaborative relationships, we create the conditions to bring out their best.

# Reference

1.    **Simms C.** How to unmask the angry patient. Am J Nurs. 1995;95:37-40.

# Chapter 7
# Pediatrics: Little People, Big Problems

*"Dr. Millard, you have to do something. Jennifer's stomach pain is not getting better and her school is demanding that she either return to classes or that we give them a letter from you explaining why she can't go to school."*

This was the third such call this week that Dr. Millard had received from Jennifer's mother, Mrs. Lyons. She felt a surge of frustration in response to the call because, after three months of trying to diagnose Jennifer's transient and migratory abdominal pain, she still did not know the cause and, worse yet, had no idea how to adequately treat it.

Jennifer presents with a common problem for pediatricians—a child with

> **Key Terms**
> - Move from expert to collaborator
> - Build a bridge with the ARCH

a chronic health problem that is difficult to diagnose and treat. Similar problems include headaches and nausea. When a child has a chronic health problem, the impact on the child's family can be significant. The child may want to stay out of school until the problem resolves, and parents may be fearful of the unknown and become excessively protective of the child, thereby limiting age-appropriate developmental activities such as school, sports, or recreational functions. Other children in the family may feel excluded. These cases can be frustrating for pediatricians because of the elusive nature of the diagnosis. At the same time, parents expect the "answer" from the pediatrician.

Jennifer's pediatrician, Stephanie Millard, has been in practice for 12 years. She became a pediatrician for the simple reason that she likes children. She has been Jennifer's doctor for nine years and has a good relationship with Jennifer and her family.

Jennifer lives with both of her parents and a five-year-old brother. Prior to the onset of her abdominal pain three months ago, she was a typical ten-year-old girl. She was involved in the local youth soccer league, attended school regularly, and was starting to learn how to play piano. Her father worked as an engineer and her mother, a grade-school teacher, stayed home to raise the children. In the past year, Mr. Lyons received a significant promotion at work that entailed being away one to three nights per week. This added stress to the family, but the additional income helped relieve some financial concerns. By all measures, the family was doing well.

When Jennifer's abdominal pain started, there was nothing remarkable occurring in the family. Initially, Jennifer's mother had called Dr. Millard's office and requested an appointment assuming that there was nothing really wrong, but she just wanted to make sure. Dr. Millard was reassuring that there did not appear to be any major problem, and that the pain should subside soon.

After a one month trial of over-the-counter antacids with no improvement, Mrs. Lyons brought Jennifer back to Dr. Millard. While Jennifer's physical exam was unchanged, her persistent pain was concerning, so Dr. Millard referred Jennifer to a gastroenterologist for further evaluation. The gastroenterologist performed a complete physical exam and decided that an endoscopy, abdominal CT, and a barium swallow test were indicated. Results of the tests suggested mild reflux and the gastroenterologist prescribed Prilosec and sent Jennifer back to Dr. Millard. Unfortunately, Jennifer's pain did not get any better.

# Step 1: Seeing the Impasse

Up until now, Dr. Millard was functioning in the role of Physician-as-Expert. She listened to Jennifer's complaints, conducted an exam, and referred her to a gastroenterologist. However, the model started to break down when Jennifer's pain did not improve. Her parents became increasingly frustrated as her attendance at school had become sporadic and she was no longer playing soccer or the piano. Jennifer was irritable and so were her parents. Dr. Millard was becoming frustrated with repeated phone calls and school excuse requests from Mrs. Lyons, yet was unsure how to proceed. The sole reliance on the Physician-as-Expert Model was leading to an impasse. Jennifer's parents requested another appointment with Dr. Millard.

# "We Need Answers"

Jennifer's mother started off the meeting with Dr. Millard with a sense of urgency.

> *"We feel like we aren't getting any answers. Sure, she has reflux, but the gastroenterologist said that the symptoms were out of proportion with the physical problem. The medicine doesn't help. It has been three months and we aren't making any progress."*

> **Mr. Lyons chimed in,** *"We need some answers. I mean, she's 10-years-old and nearly every day she has a tummy ache. That is just not normal."*

> **Dr. Millard responded,** *"I understand your frustrations. Jennifer was such a vibrant little girl and this has really thrown her off-track. She was active, doing well in school and athletics, had plenty of friends, all the things 10-year-old girls do."*

> **Mrs. Lyons agreed,** *"It really has thrown her off track. Our five-year-old son is doing so well, it's heartbreaking to see Jennifer watch life go by."*

> **Mr. Lyons pressed for an action plan.** *"We need to know what to do. What is next?"*

> *"Do you mean from a medical standpoint?"* **Dr. Millard inquired.**

> *"Yes, there has to be something else you can do to make her feel better."*

Jennifer's parents were looking externally to medicine for the answer to Jennifer's pain and her family was committed to the Physician-as-Expert-Model. Despite the fact that medicine did not have any answers, the family persisted in seeking a medical solution to the problem.

# Step 2: Understanding the Impasse

Dr. Millard felt trapped because she lacked a medical explanation for Jennifer's pain and did not know how to help her. Yet, she felt compelled to do something to help. The feeling of being trapped was the first sign of an emerging impasse. The Symptomatic Cycle (Figure 7-1) will help Dr. Millard see what is driving the impasse.

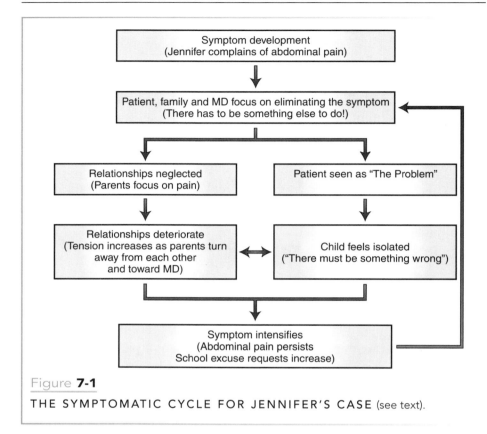

Figure **7-1**

THE SYMPTOMATIC CYCLE FOR JENNIFER'S CASE (see text).

The onset of abdominal pain starts the Symptomatic Cycle. As the pain persists, there is an increased focus on eliminating the pain, which is the obvious initial course of action. The net effect of the increased focus on eliminating the pain is that less attention gets paid to important personal relationships. That is, the relationship between Mr. and Mrs. Lyons and between them and Jennifer gets less attention as more energy is directed toward eliminating the pain. As Jennifer's pain persists, the requests for school excuses then increase.

The deterioration in relationships within the Lyons' family took several forms. When she was well, Jennifer and her father would go to the local bakery every Saturday morning for donuts. They stopped going to the bakery when, in an effort to control Jennifer's pain, fatty foods were eliminated from her diet. Jennifer and her father did not create a replacement activity for the bakery. Similarly, Jennifer and her mother routinely took long shopping trips to small boutiques in the downtown area. This activity was drastically reduced for unknown reasons.

The relationship between Mr. and Mrs. Lyons has also changed. Previously, when they had time alone, they would have romantic dates and spend a good bit of time talking about their own interests. Now, when Jennifer's father returns from business trips, the time is spent on the practicalities of running a household and arguing over how to help Jennifer. As the frustration escalates, Jennifer's parents feel increasingly powerless to help their child and the more they look to medicine for an answer, the more powerless they feel. Mrs. Lyons is feeling angry toward Mr. Lyons for his frequent travel. Mr. Lyons feels guilty about these absences and tries to take charge when he returns home.

A pattern emerged: Mr. Lyons is away, Mrs. Lyons calls him and expresses her frustration and worry about Jennifer. Mr. Lyons feels powerless, gets annoyed, and says things like: "What do you want me to do? I'm in San Francisco! Call the doctor." This creates more conflict between them and, as a result, their relationship deteriorates. Mrs. Lyons then calls Dr. Millard insisting on written excuses to keep Jennifer out of school. The family is turning to Dr. Millard for answers rather than turning toward each other in conjunction with her. The result is that each of the family members neglect parts of themselves that could potentially help Jennifer cope with her pain.

The impact of this pattern on Jennifer is that her world has shrunk around her pain. For example, in the past she talked with her friends and parents about all kinds of things including school, sports, music, and food. Now, most of Jennifer's conversations with people revolve around her pain. Her friends are calling her less often, and as the isolation increases the search for an answer to her problem intensifies.

The goal of eliminating Jennifer's pain has taken on a life of its own, and her family has put enormous amounts of energy into finding an answer that at the time did not exist. Focusing on eliminating the pain has distracted family members from the power of their relationships to help Jennifer cope with her pain. Now, let us look at how to respond to this impasse.

# Step 3. Responding to the Impasse

Jennifer's parents have become inflexible in their approach to Jennifer's pain. Consequently, this creates a blind spot by distracting them from using other skills such as limit-setting and creative problem-solving (i.e., trying half days instead of full days at school). They are so focused on turning to the expert that they have inadvertently excluded themselves from the problem-solving loop. The exclusive focus on an external solution (medicine has to have "the answer") has lead them to ignore possible internal solutions. See Box 7-1.

---

Box **7-1**

## Step 3: Responding to the Impasse

See your role in the impasse
Move from expert to collaborator
Apply the Universal Principles

---

Box **7-2**

# Universal Principles: Key Tasks for the Physician

1. Highlight competencies: "You are all doing a good job with this"
2. Focus on relationships: "We will continue to work on this together"
3. Collaborate: "Let's develop a plan together"
4. Identify each person's role and function
5 Remember to use Acceptance, Respect, Curiosity, and Honesty

Dr. Millard is at risk for developing the same blind spot as Jennifer's parents if she stays focused on the Physician-as-Expert Model of practice. Knowing her own internal signals, mainly the feelings of frustration and the urge to do something, she recognizes that it is time to shift into the Physician-as-Collaborator Model (see Figure 5-3). By moving into a collaborative mode, she will break the Symptomatic Cycle. The key task for Dr. Millard is to use the Universal Principles to build relationships with Jennifer and her family in a way that broadens their views of how to approach the problem (Box 7-2).

## Highlighting Competencies

Dr. Millard can begin the process of breaking the Symptomatic Cycle by reminding the family of skills that, up to this point, have been omitted from the problem-solving process. She does this in her next meeting with the Lyons.

Mrs. Lyons starts the meeting.

> "The longer this goes on, the harder it gets to know what to do. We (her father and I) disagree on how to deal with Jennifer's pain. I think if she is in pain, she should rest and try to feel better. He thinks she should go to school and tough it out. It has caused more than one argument in the household. He is away a good bit for work and I call him crying that I don't know what to do to help Jennifer. He gets mad at me and tells me to call you. It's hard to know what is best for her."

> **Mr. Lyons responds:** "I don't mean to disagree, but how long do we let her sit on the couch? From where I sit, we either do more tests to figure this thing out, or get on with life. I'm a busy man and I can't be spending all of this time getting nowhere."

> **Jennifer's mother continues:** "Speaking of getting on with life, Jennifer's school has had about enough of her being ab-

*sent without a clear-cut medical explanation. Could you write a blanket medical excuse for a couple of months so I don't have to be on the phone with them every day?"*

The tension and disagreement between Jennifer's parents is palpable. Dr. Millard would be fueling the tension and the Symptomatic Cycle, and then be caught in it, if she developed a blind spot like Jennifer's parents. The blind spot for Dr. Millard would be believing, like the Lyons, that medicine would provide the answer to Jennifer's pain. Focusing on a medical solution would further reinforce the parents' turning away from each other and to Dr. Millard for an answer. By ordering more tests or making minor adjustments to Jennifer's medication, she could inadvertently contribute to the Symptomatic Cycle.

Dr. Millard attempts to avoid this trap by shifting the focus of the conversation.

*"I can see this is hard on your family. At this point we have done about all of the medical tests we can—or should— do."*

*"But what if you missed something? What if it's her appendix?"* **a worried Mrs. Lyons asks.**

The tension rises as Mr. Lyons re-enters the conversation.

*"That's what she keeps saying. I say, if there is a possibility we missed something, let's go find it. So what do we do next?"*

Dr. Millard is feeling pressure to do something medical to try to help Jennifer but keeps her focus on building collaborative relationships.

*"At this point, I don't think we have missed anything. I know this is upsetting to Jennifer and your whole family. But I think the best thing to do right now is live as normal a life as possible and try to be patient. I will continue to see Jennifer as long as this continues."*

**Mr. Lyons pushes back.** *"We've been patient, but it's not getting her any better. This thing is tearing our family apart. I mean she (Jennifer) doesn't do anything but lounge around. Now she comes into our bed at night. I am starting to think she really doesn't have pain."*

*"Oh, that is just ridiculous. She is obviously in pain,"* **Mrs. Lyons shoots back.**

**Mr. Lyons pleads for help.** *"Doctor, I just don't understand why we can't figure this out. I mean, you people can cure cancer, but we can't help a 10-year-old with a stomach ache? What are we supposed to do?"*

Dr. Millard's thoughts are racing given all of the conflict and despair in the room. She feels tempted to introduce a medical option, but restrains herself and sticks to trying to highlight the competencies of Jennifer's parents.

> *"Mr. and Mrs. Lyons, I really admire your commitment to getting Jennifer well. I think both of you have been trying very hard to help Jennifer. I know you are worried that the pain could be something serious, like her appendix. I worry about that too. Mrs. Lyons, I think your worry about a stone being unturned is simply you being a protective mother. Of course you worry about that. Mr. Lyons, your thoughts about Jennifer getting on with her life are your way of wanting her to have a fulfilling life. Jennifer is lucky to have you two as her parents* (highlighted the competencies of both parents). *I have also seen Jennifer trying her best to cope with her pain. She has guts for a 10-year old. She hasn't given up on this and neither have I"* (highlights child's competencies and reinforces physician's commitment to the child and family).

> *"Thank you. It means a lot to hear someone say we're doing okay,"* a relieved Mrs. Lyons says.

Dr. Millard then shifts the conversation to being clear about her role, limits, and function.

> *"You're welcome. Given all of that, it might be helpful if we talked about what medicine can and cannot do for Jennifer."*

> Mr. Lyons agrees, *"That's why we're here today."*

# Build a Bridge with the ARCH

Dr. Millard feels like she is making progress and continues to try to build a collaborative relationship with Jennifer and her parents as an attempt to lay the groundwork for possible change.

> *"So far, Jennifer has been examined, poked, and prodded in some pretty uncomfortable ways to try to find out what is causing her pain. We have found some reflux, but nothing that fully explains her pain. I understand that you are all very frustrated by this* (Acceptance). *I admire how hard all of you are working to try to help Jennifer* (Respect). *It appears that we are looking at one of the limits of medicine right now, and I wonder if there are ways other than medical interventions that we might be able to help Jennifer* (Curiosity)? *Quite frankly, I find this frustrating, too* (Honesty)."

> Mr. Lyons responds, *"What do you mean? Like acupuncture?"*

> *"Maybe, but I think it might be helpful if we discussed how to help Jennifer live a meaningful and fulfilling life even though she has pain. Up until this point we have focused exclusively on eliminating her pain. My job is to always be thinking about medical explanations for her pain and I will never stop trying to solve that puzzle. However, if that is all we think about, we may not be using all of our resources to help her."*

> *"So, are you dumping us?"* **asked Mr. Lyons.**

> *"Absolutely not. I am Jennifer's doctor as long as you and she want me to be. But I think its time to change the way we approach her pain."*

> *"We are open to anything, but we still have to address the school issue. Can you write an excuse for her?"*

Mrs. Lyons' exasperation with the problem leads her to be open to possible change, but she remains focused on the school issue.

Mrs. Lyons' frustration and immediate concerns continue to make it difficult to broaden the approach to the problem. Dr. Millard is faced with trying to formulate a plan that will help over time and try to meet some of the family's immediate needs. Continuing to write school excuses may temporarily quell some of Mrs. Lyons' concerns, but it may paradoxically be reinforcing a narrow approach to the problem. This is a delicate balance. In order to build a collaborative relationship with the family, Dr. Millard needs to be flexible in her approach. She tries to address the issue.

> *"I understand that the school is putting pressure on you to have Jennifer return to school. I think school attendance is an important part of helping Jennifer return to a normal life."*

> *"You have to write the excuse. If you don't the school said they will start to fine us,"* **a worried Mrs. Lyons responds.**

Dr. Millard remains in a collaborative mode, but also sets limits.

> *"I didn't say I wouldn't write the excuse, but before I do, we need to agree to a plan on how to proceed."*

The conflict within the family comes out in Mr. Lyons.

> *"Well, good luck with that because we haven't been able to agree yet. I think she should be in school. Period. If there isn't anything major wrong, Jennifer needs to go to school."*

> *"I don't see how that is going to help her. She is still in pain,"* **said Mrs. Lyons.**

Dr. Millard tries to be clear about her role, limits, and function.

> "Mr. and Mrs. Lyons, it is easy to see how such a difficult problem can lead to disagreements in a family (Acceptance). As Jennifer's pediatrician, I have to keep my focus on Jennifer and her health (Defines role). Here is what I think we should do. Let's bring Jennifer in from the waiting room and include her in this discussion. If we are going to develop a plan that will work, we need her input. Can we agree on that?" (Using agreement as part of a collaborative approach.)

Dr. Millard started out simple by defining her role. By getting an agreement on a simple thing such as having Jennifer join the meeting, she is slowly shifting the focus away from the pattern of disagreements, to one of agreements. Jennifer enters the room and is greeted by Dr. Millard.

> "Hello, Jennifer, thanks for joining us. How are you today?"

> "Oh, I'm fine."

> "Good. Jennifer, your parents and I have been talking about how we might help you return to a normal life even though you are still experiencing abdominal pain. I've been impressed with how hard you have been trying to get better (highlights competency). It must be frustrating for you. One of the things we would like to try to accomplish today is to clarify how each of us can help you. I'm your pediatrician, so my job is to make sure you stay healthy. The funny thing is, that except for your abdominal pain, you are a very healthy girl."

> **Jennifer laughs and says:** "Well, that's good to know."

> "Sure it is. But we still have this problem of how to deal with your discomfort. I'm wondering what each of you can do to help Jennifer return to her life?" (Including Jennifer and her parents in the problem-solving loop.)

> "We've tried everything," **offers Mrs. Lyons.**

> "I'm not so sure about that," said Dr. Millard. "I think each of you has something to contribute here. First, besides eliminating the pain, what goal would each of you have for Jennifer right now?"

> "Go back to school" **Mr. Lyons offers definitively.**

> "Be my little girl again" **is Mrs. Lyons hope.**

> "Stop talking about this pain all the time" **a frustrated Jennifer offers.**

Dr. Millard continues to make her point.

> *"I think all of those things are possible, but not if we stay fo-cused on eliminating Jennifer's pain. Because when that is all we are thinking about, we forget to do other things."*

> *"Like what?"* **Mrs. Lyons asks.**

> *"Like talking with Jennifer about how you cope with pains that medicine has no answers to, like menstrual pain or headaches. You already know how to cope with some of life's discomforts* (highlights mothers' competency). *I'm sure Jen-nifer would be interested in what you do to help yourself. Part of life is tolerating pain. It's unfortunate, but it's true. The lesson we have been teaching Jennifer thus far is that 'when in pain, retreat from life.' Is that the message that will help her most in life?"* (Continues to highlight competencies and encourage them to become part of the collaborative process.)

> *"I think it's time to lay out each of our jobs here* (delineating role, limits, and function). *My job is to monitor Jennifer's health. Is there something really wrong with Jennifer that is causing this pain? It is unlikely, but always possible. So I would like to continue to see Jennifer once each month un-til she starts to feel better. If she gets worse, call me and I will see her sooner. In the meantime Jennifer, I will put together a health report card for you to show us that in nearly all ar-eas of your health, you are getting A's. Mr. Lyons what can your job be?"* (Helping family members start to define their roles.)

> *"I'll have to think about this one. I mean, it is easy for me to say, well you have to go to school, but that is like throwing her overboard. Jen, I really think you should be in school."*

> *"I want to go to school, but I feel like a freak if I have to raise my hand to go to the nurse's office. I'm becoming the weird kid."*

> **Mrs. Lyons tries to reassure her.** *"Well, you are not a weird kid honey. You may have a weird mother, but you are not a weird kid* (everyone laughs). *Maybe the doctor is right. It could be possible to do some of the things you used to do even though you have this pain."*

> **Mr. Lyons starts to draw on his life experience.** *"I go to work most days when my back acts up. It's not fun, but I do it."*

Dr. Millard gives the family a homework assignment intended to tap into pre-exiting competencies.

> *"I think it might help Jennifer if she had a concrete plan for what to do in school if she feels uncomfortable. Can you all talk about this, return in a few days, and let me know your plan?"*

In this exchange, Dr. Millard has highlighted the competencies of each family member and has been clear about her own limits and what role she is willing to play. Figure 7-2 illustrates how the Physician-as-Collaborator Model is being used in this scenario.

Dr. Millard continues to be vigilant in her role and function by seeking medical explanations for Jennifer's pain. When the family slowly starts to look toward each other for ways to cope with the pain by defining their roles in the process, Dr. Millard then reinforces their efforts. As part of developing a collaborative approach to the problem, the family now has a "homework assign-

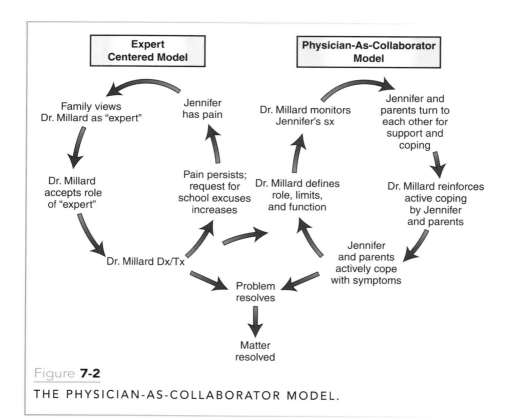

Figure **7-2**

THE PHYSICIAN-AS-COLLABORATOR MODEL.

ment." Just before the family leaves, Mrs. Lyons brings up the request for a blanket school excuse again. Here is how Dr. Millard handled it.

> *"Mrs. Lyons, I will write the school excuse for the next two days until you return to tell me about the plan your family has developed. Then we can discuss the plan and see if there is a role for school excuses."*

Dr. Millard remains in a collaborative mode by agreeing to a time-limited school excuse and demonstrated confidence in the family by saying "when you come back with a plan." The time may come when she stops writing the school excuses, but only as part of the overall plan to help Jennifer return to her life.

Three days later Jennifer and her parents returned to Dr. Millard's office. Their plan consisted of Jennifer returning to school for half-days to start. Her parents got permission for Jennifer to leave class without raising her hand to go to the nurse's office. Jennifer thought of bringing a hot-pack to school to keep in the nurses' office if she needed it. Dr. Millard agreed to write a school excuse for half-days for the next two weeks. The family was to return at that time to discuss the next steps in the plan.

# This Isn't Working

Four days later Dr. Millard received an early morning call from Jennifer's mother who was in a panic. Jennifer refused to go to school that day because of her pain and a full-day school excuse was needed right away. Dr. Millard felt her stomach tighten as the triage nurse gave her the message. Her first thought was "I thought we had solved this problem."

# Relapse Is Inevitable

Recovery from troubling or symptomatic behaviors is not linear. It occurs in fits and starts, and relapses are to be expected. The key to successfully dealing with a relapse lies in the physician's understanding of the behavior. Viewing a relapse as a failure will feed the Symptomatic Cycle. For example, if Dr. Millard viewed Jennifer's refusal to go to school as a failure in the approach being used, then she is likely to abandon the approach. The options left at that point are to set a rigid boundary ("I'm very sorry, but I will not write a full-day school excuse") or to give in and write the excuse.

With the first approach, Jennifer and her family may well feel abandoned because Dr. Millard appears to be giving up on the family. The latter approach may temporarily quell the concerns, but it will fuel the Symptomatic Cycle further leaving Dr. Millard to deal with the increasing distress. The key to success in the face of relapse is to continue to use the model of the Symptomatic Cycle to understand the problem, and then to strategically apply the universal principles to remain in a collaborative mode.

Viewing a relapse as the patient and/or family's struggle to stay on track will help move the process forward. Here is how Dr. Millard applied this principle in Jennifer's case when she returns Mrs. Lyons call.

> "Good morning, Mrs. Lyons. I got your message. Can you tell me what is happening?"
>
> "Yes, Jennifer says her stomach really hurts today and she won't go to school, so I need a full-day excuse from you."

Dr. Millard feels annoyed at the immediate request for a school excuse, but contains her emotions.

> "Well, let's back up to our talk a few days ago. If I recall, the plan was for Jennifer to go to school for half-days for two weeks and then we would re-evaluate."
>
> "That's right, but she is refusing to go to school today. I know the school will start to fine us if we don't provide a medical excuse."
>
> "Okay, first, I think it's good that Jennifer has been able to go school for half-days for at least a couple of days. I think you can take some comfort that Jennifer and you and her dad are making progress (Highlights competencies). Have you spoken with her dad about this?" (Tries to decrease mother's isolation.)
>
> "Well, no, not yet. I just thought I had to get the full-day school excuse first." Mrs. Lyons is reverting to the old way of dealing with the problem. This is the re-emergence of the Symptomatic Cycle. Dr. Millard remains patient and stays the course.
>
> "I understand your concern (Accepts mother's position that the school excuse is important). Mrs. Lyons, you have been making great progress in helping Jennifer cope with her pain and function more effectively (Highlights competence again). Here is what I think we should do (Deliberately uses the word "we" to convey a collaborative approach to the dilemma). Why don't you call your husband and discuss this? Then, if you two agree that Jennifer should stay out of school for the entire day, I will see her later this morning to evaluate her pain."

Dr. Millard is decreasing Mrs. Lyons isolation by encouraging her to share the problem with her husband and by offering to see Jennifer later that morning. She is also avoiding becoming caught in the Symptomatic Cycle by continuing to use a framework that encourages the emergence of the competencies of Jennifer and her parents. Finally, she is sending a clear message that she will work with Jennifer and her parents. She is not passing judgment, nor is she giving up. The message she is sending is that "we" will continue to work on this, and by doing so, she is holding herself, and everyone else, accountable to their agreement.

An hour later, Jennifer's mother called the office to report that Jennifer was feeling a bit better and would go to school that afternoon.

## Scenario Resolution

After about nine weeks Jennifer returned to school full-time. During that time her mother's calls to Dr. Millard slowly decreased. There were two days when Jennifer refused to go to school and Dr. Millard saw her. Though her physical exam was unremarkable, she wrote a full-day excuse. When she did write the excuse, she reminded Jennifer and her parents that they were indeed making progress and she had complete faith in their ability to continue to do so. Jennifer gradually returned to playing sports and the piano as her abdominal pain was no longer the focus of her life. She is now seen by Dr. Millard for periodic check-ups and occasional illnesses.

## Practice Points

Dealing with the uncertainty of some medical problems requires patience and persistence. Amid the uncertainty, there are a few points that may be helpful:

1. **Be true to yourself.** Let your integrity and principles guide you through periods of uncertainty.

2. **Include patients and families in the problem-solving process.** A good way to help people mobilize their internal resources is to include them in the process of trying to find ways to cope with the ongoing medical problems.

3. **Expect relapses to occur.** The push for change may trigger a return to troubling behaviors by patients and family members. This is a sign of their ongoing struggle to adapt to the adversity they are facing. Even though it may feel like a failure ("Here we go again."), focusing on developing collaborative relationships will help you to stay the course and avoid the impulse to abandon ship.

# Chapter 8

# "You Have to Save My Little Girl!": Crisis in the Intensive Care Unit

## "I Believe in Miracles"

Maria Thomas, an 18-year-old, was admitted to the Intensive Care Unit (ICU) at 2 a.m. after being rescued from a house fire by firefighters. Her case is not unusual in that it revolved around family members, one of whom was emotionally volatile, disagreeing on the appropriate course of medical care. During the fire, she suffered severe anoxic and ischemic injuries to her brain, and it appeared that Maria was progressing toward brain death.

At the time of the fire, Maria was at home caring for three younger siblings.

**Key Terms**

- Safety first
- Highlight competencies
- Decrease isolation and disconnection

Maria's parents' divorced six years ago, and she was living with her mother and step-father, who were at a local bar when the fire occurred. Maria has had limited contact with her father for the past six years. But he came to the ICU after hearing about the fire, and when he arrived, he was grief-stricken and began yelling;

> *"You have to do more to save my little girl. I believe in the*
> *Lord! I believe in miracles! You can't let her die!"*

When Maria arrived in the emergency room, a complete work-up including an MRI of her brain and chest x-ray showed the extent of her injuries. She was intubated and transferred to the ICU within a matter of hours of her arrival at the hospital. With each passing hour her intracranial pressure rose, causing concern that Maria's brain would herniate, causing brain death. While the ICU team believed that everything possible was being done to save Maria's life, her attending physician believed that she would soon die from her injuries.

Maria's attending physician is Frank Graham. He has been working in intensive care units for 18 years. He is calm and meticulous and is considered by his colleagues to be gifted in his ability to deal with challenging cases. That gift was about to be tested.

Dr. Graham felt that Maria was stable, yet very critical as he left the ICU to meet with her parents. When he met them in the hallway, he introduced himself and extended his hand. Mr. Thomas turned away. Mrs. Rourke, Maria's mother, greeted him and asked if her spouse could join them. Dr. Graham paused briefly, then agreed. He invited the three people into a small conference room to give them the grim news about Maria. As soon as he entered the room, he realized he had made a mistake. By agreeing to have Mrs. Rourke's spouse join them, the room felt lopsided. Given Mr. Thomas's defensiveness, he seemed outnumbered in the room. Dr. Graham noticed this but since he had already agreed that Maria's step-father could be present, he did not now want to ask him to leave, so he proceeded with the meeting.

> *"First, I just want to say how sorry I am about this tragedy."*

Mrs. Rourke thanked him for his concern while Mr. Thomas paced frantically around the room and demanded:

> *"What do you mean tragedy? What is going on here?"*
>
> *"Mr. Thomas, I will get to that. Why don't you sit down so we*
> *can talk about Maria's condition?"*
>
> *"Don't tell me what to do! What is going on with my daugh-*
> ter?"* **Mr. Thomas responded angrily.**

Dr. Graham was surprised by the intense anger in Mr. Thomas' voice but proceeded with his explanation of Maria's medical condition.

*"When Maria was in the fire several things happened to her. She inhaled a lot of smoke and hot gases which hurt her lungs. Her brain was also starved of oxygen for some period of time. When this happens to a person's brain, the cells in the brain actually die. The brain is different from other parts of our body in that when cells in a person's brain die, they do not regenerate. This is unlike, say your skin. If you get a cut, you bleed, develop a scab, and eventually the skin heals itself. You may have a scar, but there is healing. The brain cannot do that."*

*"So what does this mean,"* asked Mrs. Rourke?

*"Right now, Maria's brain is so injured that it is swelling. As it continues to swell, it is putting a lot of pressure on the inside of her skull. We are trying very hard to control that swelling, but as of right now, we cannot. If this goes on, Maria will most likely not survive her injuries."*

**In tears, Mrs. Rourke asks:** *"Is there anything else that can be done?"*

*"We're doing everything possible."*

**Mr. Thomas explodes.** *"Bull____! That's what I say— bull____! What do you mean you are doing everything possible? You're giving up, that's what you are doing. She has only been here a few hours, how can you be talking about her dying already?"*

*"Mr. Thomas, I am being as honest as I can with you,"* a stunned Dr. Graham responds.

*"There's a problem here doctor. You know what it is? I'll tell you what it is. You are not a man of faith. Because if you were a man of faith, you would be praying with us and speaking the hopeful message of our Lord and savior Jesus Christ!"*

# Physician-as-Expert

The model of Physician-as-Expert is important, but limited, in Maria's case. In addition to the medical expertise necessary to address Maria's acute and critical problems, Dr. Graham needs a strong set of skills to deal with Mr. Thomas.

Dr. Graham feels overwhelmed by Mr. Thomas' anger. He tried to be clear and compassionate in telling Maria's parents the dismal prognosis, but the intensity of Mr. Thomas' response disoriented even this experienced physician. Unsure of how to proceed, he suggests that they all meet in a few hours to further discuss Maria's medical status. Dr. Graham then returns to the ICU and is met by the clinical head nurse

> *"We have a real problem with Maria Thomas' father. He is ranting and raving in the room. When the night shift nurse asked him to calm down, he said that he was calm. He then said 'You don't want to see me get mad.' He is being abusive toward the nurses and is disturbing other families in the ICU. What can we do?"*

Dr. Graham feels anger building up and instructs the head nurse to "Tell your nurses that if he gets out of line again, they should call security."

Dr. Graham feels increasing anger because in addition to having 14 other critically ill patients to attend to, the nurses are feeling frightened and are looking for him to "fix the problem." In response, he suggested they call security. Here is how the interaction went when a nurse followed Dr. Graham's advice.

> *"Mr. Thomas, your behavior has been very disruptive to the nurses and the other families on this unit. If you don't maintain some sense of control, we will be forced to call security."*
>
> *"Security? Those rent-a-cops! They don't scare me—I've been to jail, lady."*

# Step 1: Seeing the Impasse

The threat of calling security has only increased Mr. Thomas' aggressive statements. The efforts to get him to calm down are paradoxically contributing to an escalation in his behavior. An impasse has arrived. But what is driving this dilemma? The Symptomatic Cycle will help us to understand the dynamics that are fueling this impasse.

# Step 2: Understanding the Impasse

Figure 8-1 illustrates this impasse in the model of the Symptomatic Cycle.

As Mr. Thomas continues to make threatening statements, staff members become more frightened and act on their fear by threatening to call security. This attempt to impose control backfires, and Mr. Thomas becomes increasingly threatening. This leads staff to try once again to "get him to calm down." The harder the staff try to gain a sense of control, the more Mr. Thomas lets them know that he will not be controlled.

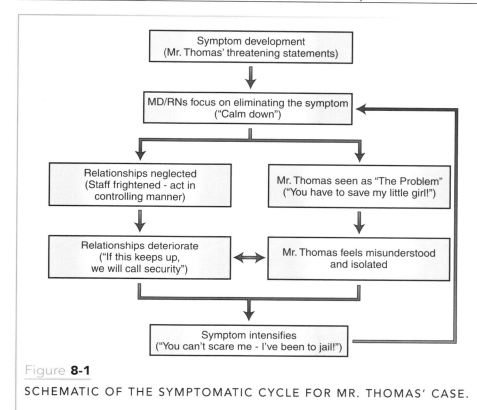

Figure **8-1**

SCHEMATIC OF THE SYMPTOMATIC CYCLE FOR MR. THOMAS' CASE.

This type of case is particularly difficult because people feel threatened by Mr. Thomas. The nurses and physicians do not know if he has a history of violence, but by his behavior and report of being in jail, he might be capable of violence. When staff members are frightened, the first step in developing a plan to resolve the impasse must address safety and security issues. But how can that be done when the threats of calling security are only escalating the troubling behavior?

# Step 3: Responding to the Impasse

The first step in breaking the Symptomatic Cycle is to address the staff's safety concerns. While the impulse in this case is to get Mr. Thomas to calm down, focusing exclusively on that goal will create a blind spot for staff. The blind spot will be that the staff's fear will result in them ignoring their own interpersonal competencies, thereby acting defensively toward Mr. Thomas. This could then contribute to an escalation in Mr. Thomas' behavior. Dr. Graham

---

Box **8-1**

# Responding to the Impasse. Key Tasks for the Physician

1. Safety first
2. Highlight their competencies
3. Decrease the isolation and disconnection of staff members and Mr. Thomas by focusing on relationships (Use the ARCH)
4. Move from control to collaboration

---

decided that his framework for trying to diffuse this situation would be to decrease the isolation and disconnection of the nurses and Mr. Thomas by first highlighting their respective competencies. Since the safety issues were paramount, he began by meeting with the clinical head nurse and the nurse who was caring for Maria. See Box 8-1.

# Safety First

*"Thanks for taking the time to talk about this case. First, I want to thank you for being involved. I know Mr. Thomas' behavior is very disturbing. I was just back with Maria and she is getting outstanding nursing care. It is impressive that you are able to stay focused on her care even though her father is so distracting (Highlight competence)."*

One of Maria's nurses commented, *"Thanks, but it is not easy. He is ranting and raving and keeps saying that there is going to be some miracle. He also says we can't let her die and he seems really angry when he says that. He's totally in denial."*

The head nurse was clear in her assessment. *"I think he is a threat. He is a bully and the nurses are scared of him."*

Dr. Graham asked, *"Are you scared of him?"*

The floor nurse responded, *"Well, yes. I just don't know what he is going to do next. I am worried that he is going to attack me or come in with a gun or something crazy."*

*"We can't have that. You have to feel safe,"* a concerned Dr. Graham said.

*"Yes, but when I told him we would call security, he really went off."*

*"I heard. That was my mistake. I was upset about having to spend so much time on this case and hoped that the threat of calling security would be enough to calm him down. Anyway, we have to develop a plan to help you feel safe and keep your attention on caring for Maria. I believe it would be helpful to have two nurses assigned to Maria's care. My idea is that no nurse would ever be alone in the room at any time (Attempt to decrease their isolation). What do you think?"*

*"I don't know. We are so busy, I really don't want to be a burden to other nurses."*

**The head nurse also expressed concern,** *"I like the idea, but how can we do that? We are at capacity and I don't have any nurses to spare."*

**Dr. Graham took a leadership role.** *"Call another nurse to come in."*

*"I am not sure I can. Administration has been giving me a hard time about the over-time pay in the unit."*

**Graham offers to intervene.** *"I will talk to the people in administration if they give you a hard time (Decreases head nurse's isolation by offering to take the blame for a potential budget problem). We just need to do this. Finally, if any of the nurses feel directly threatened, tell them to leave the room and call security. We can't take any chances with your safety."*

Dr. Graham's first step was to decrease the isolation of the nursing staff, which in turn, may help them feel safe. He instructed the nurses to use their existing supports, and if necessary, to page him if they were scared or had any concerns about Maria's care or Mr. Thomas' behavior. He also spoke directly to them, or had one of the residents speak to them, regularly throughout the day. The next step in the process was to attempt to develop a more productive relationship with Mr. Thomas.

# Highlight Competencies

Dr. Graham's framework for interrupting the Symptomatic Cycle is to use the Physician-as-Collaborator Model and to apply the ARCH principles (Acceptance, Respect, Curiosity, and Honesty) to develop a better relationship with Mr. Thomas. Acceptance of a person who is angry and threatening is a difficult task. Trying to find something—anything—he liked about Mr. Thomas was Dr. Graham's first goal. He would also attempt to highlight some of Mr. Thomas' competencies. Dr. Graham was hopeful that if he could start to build a relationship with Mr. Thomas, then his disruptive behavior would dissipate. Here is how the meeting with Mr. Thomas went.

> *"Thank you for agreeing to meet with me Mr. Thomas."*
>
> *"I need some answers about Maria. Are you people going to fight for her or not?"*
>
> *Dr. Graham controls his impulse to lash out at Mr. Thomas. "I admire how hard you are fighting for Maria (Highlight competency). We are fighting for her too."*
>
> *"Then why do I hear the nurses talking about brain death, whatever that is?"*
>
> *"Brain death is a medical term that..."*

Dr. Graham catches himself reverting to the Physician-as-Expert Model of trying to convince Mr. Thomas of Maria's poor medical prognosis. He changes course and tries to focus on building a collaborative relationship with Mr. Thomas.

> *"Before we get into all of the medical stuff, would you tell me a little bit about Maria (Curiosity)? I can tell by how passionately you are trying to protect her (Highlight competence) that she means a lot to you."*
>
> *"She is a good girl. She didn't deserve this. I cannot understand what in the world she was doing at home, alone, at two in the morning caring for all of those kids while that witch was out getting drunk with her no-good husband. Does that make any sense to you?"*
>
> *"This is a real tragedy."*
>
> *"I can tell you this, when this is all over, I am going to take care of some business."*

Dr. Graham feels a degree of threat and considers telling Mr. Thomas that security will be called if he gets out of hand, but decides to refocus on the relationship first.

> *"Mr. Thomas, I cannot imagine how upsetting this must be for you (Acceptance)."*
>
> *"You're darn right it is."*
>
> *"Given how hard this must be for you, I appreciate that you are here for Maria and that you are fighting for her interests (Continues to highlight competency)."*

*"From where I sit, it doesn't look like anyone else is."*

Dr. Graham is annoyed at the implication that staff are not acting in Maria's interest. He contains his annoyance and considers his options. He feels like he is too annoyed to continue with this meeting and does not know what to do next, so he asks to meet later.

*"With your permission, could we meet in a few hours to continue to discuss Maria's medical condition? Would you be willing to do that?"*

Dr. Graham asks for his agreement to meet in an effort to move away from a controlling statement—"We need to meet again in two hours"—and toward a collaborative mode. Mr. Thomas agrees, but not without some irritation.

*"I'll be here. I am not going to leave her alone."*

# Decrease Isolation

Dr. Graham thought he had done a decent job of trying to build a relationship with Mr. Thomas, even though he continued to be abrasive. Graham returned to the ICU to care for his other patients.

Two hours later Dr. Graham was notified that the consulting neurologist had performed an exam and determined that Maria was brain dead. The hospital policy on brain death mandated that a second brain death exam be performed within six hours of the first exam to confirm the findings. The news circulated around the ICU quickly and staff began having hallway conversations about the issue of withdrawing ventilatory support from Maria.

# A Crisis Looms

Dr. Graham knew that a potential crisis could emerge if Mr. Thomas continued to believe that Maria would recover. The likelihood that Mr. Thomas would agree to removing life-support technology seemed small if this belief persisted. The clinical head nurse approached Dr. Graham and asked him what he planned to do if Mr. Thomas refused to agree to withdraw life-support. Dr. Graham felt a flash of anger but contained himself. The anger was driven by a sense of powerlessness over how to deal with Mr. Thomas. Dr. Graham continued to think of the universal principles as a guide for responding in a collaborative manner. He suggested a meeting with the nurses to address their concerns.

**Dr. Graham:** *So, neurology says she meets brain death criteria. How are things going in the room?*

**RN:** *About the same. Mr. Thomas keeps saying a miracle is coming. He even alluded to us not knowing what we are doing.*

**Head Nurse (HN):** *What if Mr. Thomas is still in denial after the second brain death exam is done?*

**Dr. Graham:** *I am not sure. Technically, we don't need his permission to withdraw support. Brain death is death. If she is brain dead, we can withdraw life-support. But I don't think we should do that because it will probably set him off.*

**RN:** *The nurses feel like we are caring for a corpse. I mean, she is dead and we are keeping the ventilator going just because of her father. Why can't we just turn it off after the second brain death exam?*

**Dr. Graham:** *Let's cross that bridge later. For right now, the first question is, are the nurses feeling any safer?*

**RN:** *Yes, having someone else in the room helps me stay focused on her care and I think Mr. Thomas is less aggressive with two nurses in there.*

**Dr. Graham:** *I am meeting with him again shortly. I think someone from nursing should be present.*

Dr. Graham was including the nurses in the discussion as a way of further decreasing their isolation.

# Provocative Parent

Dr. Graham and the clinical head nurse then meet with Mr. Thomas and Mrs. Rourke. Dr. Graham's goal is to remain respectful and to highlight competencies whenever possible:

*"How are each of you doing?"*

Mrs. Rourke was eager for information.

*"We just need to know what is happening with Maria. We heard one of the doctors say something about brain death."*

**Mr. Thomas says,** *"I don't think you people know what you are doing. How could she be brain dead? Have you seen her? She is breathing and her skin is warm. Last I knew dead people didn't breathe and they were cold! I think we need to get her to a hospital where the doctors know what they are doing."*

Dr. Graham feels another flash of anger toward Mr. Thomas in response to his provocative statements. If he responds to this, he will be caught in the Symptomatic Cycle, so he pauses and remembers the universal principles.

*"Mr. Thomas, I respect your commitment to getting Maria the best possible medical care (Respect and highlights competency). Would it help if I explained what is happening with Maria?"(Curiosity)*

*"I guess so."*

*"The term you have heard, brain death, means that Maria's brain has stopped functioning in a way that can support life. Mr. Thomas, you are correct that she is warm and appears to be breathing (Highlights competency). That's because we are using machines to keep her lungs working and blood circulating throughout her body. Without those machines, she will stop breathing and her heart will stop."*

*"So keep the machines going until we can find a real doctor who can help her."*

**Dr. Graham remains composed.** *"The way the determination of brain death works is that a neurologist has to perform two separate exams, about six hours apart, before a final declaration is made. The first exam was done and the second one will happen in a few hours. During that time, we will keep the machines going. After the next exam we will have to have a discussion about the findings. I fully expect that the second exam will confirm that Maria is brain dead."*

*"Then we need to get her to another hospital that will not pull the plug. I know the Lord will save my little girl! You people do not have enough faith that the good Lord will perform a miracle."*

Dr. Graham feels increasingly annoyed but sticks to his framework of trying to build a relationship with Mr. Thomas.

*"Mr. Thomas, if you would like Maria transferred to another hospital, we will do that. I know you love her and only want what is best for her (Highlight competency). It will be up to you to find a hospital that will care for her. If you do, we will do everything we can to get her transferred. Is there anything else we can do for either of you right now?"*

Mr. Thomas is a bit surprised by Dr. Graham's response.

*"Like what?"*

*"Well, Mr. Thomas, you are a very religious man and if there is someone from your church, a pastor perhaps, who we could call and ask to come in and pray with you, we would be happy to do that."*

*"I do not belong to a church. I do not need a fancy building to worship the Almighty."*

*"In that case, we have chaplains here in the hospital who could come and pray with you. Would you like us to contact them?"*

*"That would be fine. Tell them to bring along the good book."*

In this interaction, Dr. Graham contained his frustration and anger in response to Mr. Thomas' provocative statements. By keeping the universal principles in mind, he avoided any escalation in Mr. Thomas' behavior. The conflict over withdrawing life-support was not resolved, but Dr. Graham has accomplished the goals of slowly developing a collaborative relationship with Mr. Thomas and helping the nurses feel less isolated.

## "She's Brain Dead. Now What?"

Several hours later, the neurologist returned to the ICU and performed a second brain death exam. The findings were consistent with the first exam; Maria was brain dead. The clinical head nurse approaches Dr. Graham.

HN: *She's brain dead. Now what?*

**Dr. Graham:** *Well, I suppose we have to start the organ procurement process.*

HN: *Oh no, he is going to lose it if he is approached about donating her organs.*

**Dr. Graham:** (Sighs) *Let's start by meeting with her parents and telling them that brain death has been confirmed and see what happens.*

Dr. Graham and the clinical head nurse meet again with Maria's parents. Dr. Graham starts the meeting.

*"I am very sorry, but the second brain death exam has confirmed the findings of the first exam. Maria is brain dead."*

Mrs. Rourke starts to sob and Mr. Thomas paces frantically across the room. Mr. Thomas starts to shake.

*"I knew it. You just want to get her out of here. (Holds up a bible) You will have to answer to your creator!"*

**The head nurse tries to be empathic.** *"Mr. Thomas, we are truly sorry for your loss."*

*"What loss? She is not dead!"*

Dr. Graham knows that the interaction is stuck and that he needs to do something to try to move it forward. He decides to take a risk and be honest with Mr. Thomas.

*"Sir, may I ask you something (Respect and curiosity)?"*

*"What?"*

*"Mr. Thomas, I know you are a man of great faith and that you are trying as hard as you can to do what is right for your daughter (highlights competencies). But, how do you expect us (points to the head nurse) to take care of your beautiful daughter if you are scaring the hell out of us (honesty)?"*

**Mr. Thomas looks stunned.** *"What?"*

**Dr. Graham continues,** *"Sir, we are frightened of you (honesty). And if we are scared of you, it takes our attention away from Maria. I know we all want Maria to get the best care possible but we can't do that if we are frightened of you."*

**Mrs. Rourke chimes in,** *"He is like this with everyone."*

**Mr. Thomas sits down.** *"I am not trying to scare you. I just don't want to lose her."*

**Dr. Graham continues,** *"Of course you don't want to lose her. We know you are trying to be a good father when she needs you the most (Highlight competency). But right now, we are out of miracles. Maybe the Lord will intervene, but so far, it hasn't happened. It might help us to take better care of Maria, if you could tell us how we can help you right now (Curiosity)?"*

*"I need time."*

*"Okay, how much?"*

*"I need time to make some things right."*

*"Can we help you?"*

*"I don't know if I can trust you."*

**Dr. Graham remains curious.** *"Can you tell us a little more?"*

**Mr. Thomas is hesitant, but goes on:** *"Maria has a half-sister. They didn't see each other a lot, but when they did they really got along well. Her half-sister is only 14 so she can't drive here. I think they should see each other."*

*"Where does she live?"*

*"About an hour from here. I could go get her, but I don't know if you guys will pull the plug before I return."*

**Dr. Graham sees an opportunity,** *"I will give you my word that we will not withdraw support before you return. I trust you sir (Respect). I know you want to do something good for Maria right now. This is your chance. I will wait. (Stands up and extends his hand.) Do I have your word that you will return?"*

**Mr. Thomas stands up and shakes Dr. Graham's hand.** *"Yes."*

# Scenario Resolution

Mr. Thomas left the hospital to get Maria's half-sister. Staff members were anxious that he would not return. After three hours, they began to ask Dr. Graham how long he would give Mr. Thomas to return. Dr. Graham admitted that he did not know. He continued to emphasize that the nurses were giving Maria outstanding care and that they were contributing to her dignified death.

After four hours, Mr. Thomas returned to the hospital with Maria's half-sister and they both visited Maria. The organ procurement staff then asked to speak with Maria's mother and father. The nurses and Dr. Graham expected Mr. Thomas to explode, but he agreed to the meeting. Both parents ultimately agreed to donate some of Maria's organs for transplantation. She was taken to the operating room where mechanical ventilation was removed and she stopped breathing almost immediately with both parents by her side.

The next morning, Mr. Thomas returned to the ICU. The ICU staff were hesitant and a bit frightened when they first saw him. But his mission was simple; he found the head nurse and Dr. Graham and with tears in his eyes said, "Thanks for putting up with me."

## Summary

This case shows the importance of remaining connected to others, colleagues and patients, even when it is hard to do so. The intense feelings generated by similar cases (uncertainty, fear, and even anger) are difficult to tolerate alone. Reaching out to colleagues and finding helpful ways to relate to patients and family members under these circumstances are good ways to find creative solutions to seemingly impossible problems.

# Practice Points

1. **Tolerate feelings.** Tolerating intense feelings, regardless of how unpleasant they may be, will help the other person to feel accepted and understood. When people feel accepted and understood, they are more likely to be open to change.

2. **Don't go it alone.** Intense feelings in clinical encounters can distract you from the task at hand. Asking a colleague to join you during the encounter can be an easy way to decrease your own isolation and keep you focused.

3. **Honesty pays.** Respectfully and sensitively letting patients know what you need and where your limits are, sets the stage for a collaborative relationship.

# Chapter 9
# Ethical Dilemmas in Medicine (Or are They?)*

Barbara Peterson is 23 years old and was recently diagnosed with metastatic sarcoma. She was admitted to the intensive care unit of a large urban hospital five days earlier in septic shock. Although the acute crisis has resolved, her mood has become sullen and withdrawn, except for when she asks members of the medical staff to help her die. At those times she perks up and makes provocative statements such as "What's the quickest way to die? How many of these pills do I need to kill myself?" The members of the staff are uncomfortable with the requests, yet do not know how to respond to her or help her.

> **Key Terms**
>
> - Breaking the cycle: from helpless to hopeful
> - You always have something to offer

# Moral Guidance

This scenario raises a number of important issues relevant to the care of terminally ill patients. Foremost is how to deal with requests for assisted death (1-2). One aspect of the issue is the moral concern of whether physicians and other health care providers should aid a patient who requests help with dying. These moral concerns can be addressed by using the traditional methods of bioethics, which include fact gathering, determining competency, delineating ethical issues and competing ethical claims, then moving toward resolution (3).

But sometimes the moral issues are secondary, such as when requests for assisted suicide are not really genuine expressions of a wish to die, but instead are about something altogether different, such as a conflict in relationships or a breakdown in effective communication. In these situations, the compelling nature of life-and-death situations can so impair communication that people are distracted by the "ethics" to the exclusion of the relationships. Then, the traditional approaches to resolving ethical dilemmas in medicine are less helpful because their narrow focus on normative issues provides little guidance for addressing the impasse in relationships. Since ethical conflicts in medicine are often laced with such interpersonal dimensions, they can benefit from broader approaches that explicitly address the interpersonal aspects of ethical dilemmas. Our models will help the staff and Ms. Peterson find a way to deal with her requests for death.

# "What's the Quickest Way to Die?"

Two years prior to this hospitalization, Ms. Peterson had a sarcoma surgically removed from her left thigh. She was feeling well until four weeks earlier, when she developed night sweats and difficulty breathing. When her symptoms appeared, Ms. Peterson was engaged to be married and was preparing to graduate from college.

Highly intelligent and an accomplished collegiate athlete, Ms. Peterson was a natural leader on her college campus. Her family described her as open and approachable, and part of a tight-knit family who were always able to "talk things out." Ms. Peterson's mother describes the change she saw in her daughter when the sarcoma recurred:

> "Barbara was always a person who would talk about difficult things. At college, her friends and teammates would go to her when they had problems and she would listen and try to help them. She was a high-energy person who didn't let things get her down. Until this. Now, it seems like she is in another world. She hardly speaks to any of us and when she does, quite frankly, the things she says are so upsetting that we don't know what to say in response. So we just keep our mouths closed. I feel like she is drifting away."

Barbara's mother was not alone in her frustrations. Justin Blake is a critical care fellow who is taking care of Ms. Peterson. He is in the second year of his fellowship and has seen many difficult cases. He talks about his initial interactions with Ms. Peterson.

> *"When she was first admitted to the hospital, I told her that there was no cure for her disease. She was quiet, but seemed to be okay. I also told her that we could offer her palliative care to treat her symptoms and to help keep her comfortable. Again, no response. I figured she was just in shock and trying to absorb some pretty terrible news. I had no idea she would become such a problem."*

The first sign of trouble came when a nurse went into Ms. Peterson's room to give her pain medicine. As the nurse was administering the medicine Ms. Peterson said:

> *"How many of these pills do I need to take to kill myself?"*
> *The nurse was stunned and said, "Don't talk like that."*

Later that day Dr. Blake went in to see Ms. Peterson and had a similar interaction.

> *"Good morning Ms. Peterson, how are you feeling today?"*

After a minute with no response, Dr. Blake continued with his routine.

> *"Can I listen to your lungs?"*

Ms. Peterson continued to be silent so Dr. Blake proceeded with his exam.

> *"Ok, it will only take a moment. My stethoscope might be a little cold."*

Ms. Peterson finally breaks the silence.

> *"How come no one will tell me how many of those white pills I need to take to kill myself?"*

Dr. Blake is flustered by the question and responds,

> *"Well, you know that it's against the law for doctors to help patients die."*

> *"At this point, do you really think I care about the law?"*

> *"Probably not."*

Disoriented and angry, Dr. Blake said he had to answer a page and left the room. This interaction became typical; Ms. Peterson would be quiet and then suddenly make a provocative statement. Some of the staff felt ambushed by her behavior and would leave the room feeling flustered and angry.

A few days later, Dr. Blake was in Ms. Peterson's room when out of the blue she said,

> *"Can you give me enough medicine to end this? What's the quickest way to die?"*

Dr. Blake did not know how to respond.

Ms. Peterson continued to make spontaneous requests for death. The ICU staff, while moved by her plight, were uncomfortable with her requests and tried hard to get her to stop making such disturbing statements. Her primary nurse described her strategy.

> "When I go into her room, I take one of two paths. I either go in as quiet as possible and hang the bag and run, or I just talk non-stop while I am in there. That way she really can't enter the conversation. I feel bad, but it helps keep her crazy statements to a minimum. One thing is for sure, I am not going to help kill her."

Other nurses, and some physicians, reported that they tried to avoid going into Ms. Peterson's room. While they felt guilty for using this tactic, they did not see any other options. Despite all of the efforts to avoid Ms. Peterson and her disturbing statements, things were about to get worse.

# Step 1: Seeing the Impasse

As Ms. Peterson's requests for assisted death escalated, the ICU staff became increasingly frustrated; they felt powerless to change her condition and were frightened by her statements. The case reached a crisis point one morning when Dr. Blake entered Ms. Peterson's room and found her sitting up in bed with her eyes closed. She was ashen-looking and had a nasal cannula delivering oxygen. She appeared to be air hungry and her speech was barely audible. Her mother and brother stood in a corner of the room with their arms folded. Ms. Peterson motioned for Dr. Blake to come closer and whispered,

> "Will you please shoot me tonight?"

Dr. Blake's head snapped back in response to the graphic nature of her request. It was as if someone had punched him in the forehead. He talks about that morning.

> "It was just another busy morning on rounds and then, wham, she asks me to shoot her. If she hadn't been so polite about it, I probably would have yelled at her. For a second I thought maybe she was encepholopathic, because who in their right mind asks a doctor to shoot them? Finally I said 'I can't do that.' She then laid her head back on her pillow and closed her eyes. The conversation was over."

When word of this incident circulated throughout the ICU, there was a marked turn in people's attitudes toward Ms. Peterson. Her primary nurse describes the shift.

*"When we heard about what she said to Justin, people flipped. Who does she think she is talking to a doctor like that? The feeling was that she had crossed the line into completely unacceptable territory. It is one thing to ask how much morphine it takes to kill some one. It is another thing entirely to ask a physician to pull the trigger."*

The relationship between Ms. Peterson and her caregivers had reached a critical point with her latest request for death. The staff was angry at her and were on the verge of imposing more controls in an effort to eliminate her disturbing statements. Of course, further attempts to impose controls would paradoxically increase the disturbing statements. The impasse had arrived.

# Step 2: Understanding the Impasse

The Symptomatic Cycle can be used to help visualize and understand the impasse between Ms. Peterson and her caregivers (Figure 9-1).

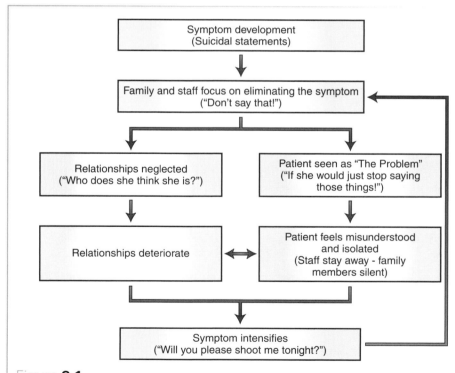

Figure **9-1**

SCHEMATIC OF THE SYMPTOMATIC CYCLE IN MS. PETERSON'S CASE (see text).

The "symptoms" were her suicidal statements and requests for staff assistance in her death. As Ms. Peterson's family and the medical staff tried to get her to stop making such provocative statements about death, Ms. Peterson became more withdrawn, which contributed to her isolation. Medical staff unintentionally contributed to her isolation by avoiding her room, and family members became silent because they did not know how to respond to her. As her statements became more graphic and forceful, Ms. Peterson became increasingly isolated because no one wanted to be around her. This pattern was frustrating for the ICU staff because they believed they were doing all they could to be helpful to Ms. Peterson and her family. Yet, when their efforts were met with anger, hostility, or opposition, staff members withdrew further, thereby cementing the impasse.

# See Your Role in the Impasse

Dr. Blake was stuck and he knew it. He shared his frustration with a couple of colleagues in the on-call room. (See Box 9-1).

> *"This case is driving me crazy. What kind of person asks their doctor to shoot them? I mean, does she really think I would do that?"*

One of Dr. Blake's colleagues, Dr. Powers, replies,

> *"No way. She is pushing your buttons, man."*

> *"She is pushing my buttons! The question is, how do I get her to stop?"*

> *"Push back."*

> *"I tried that, but is doesn't work. The more we try to get her to stop saying those crazy things, the more she says them. Honestly, the minute I go into her room all I want to do is run out of there."*

> **Dr. Powers challenges him,** *"Maybe that is part of the problem?"*

---

Box **9-1**

## Applying the Universal Principles:

1. See your role in the impasse
2. Focus on relationships
3. Be clear about your role, limits, and function
4. Use the ARCH

*"What do you mean? I'm working super hard on this case."*

*"I'm sure you are, but I know that when I get cases like this, my impulse is to flee too. After a couple of my own disasters, a few wise attendings taught me, well, maybe hammered into my head, that if you try to suspend judgment and listen a bit closer, you might actually get to the bottom of the problem."*

*"I don't need an amateur shrink right now."*

*"I agree. It sounds more like you need a professional."*

Dr. Blake was desperate and as much as he did not want to admit it, he thought that Dr. Powers had made a good point. Perhaps if he took a different approach to Ms. Peterson, things might go in a different direction. Ironically, Ms. Peterson's provocative statements were driving people away at a critical time when what she most needed was to have people close to her. He would have to find a way to get closer to her. This is when applying the universal principles could help him to transition from the role of expert to one of collaborator (Figure 9-2).

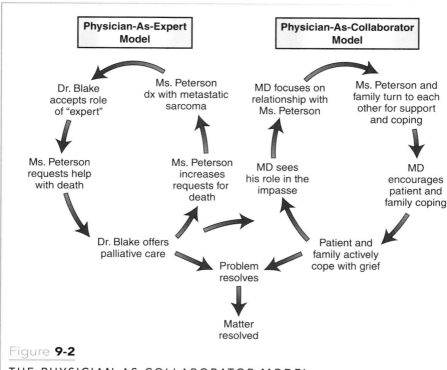

Figure **9-2**

THE PHYSICIAN-AS-COLLABORATOR MODEL.

His plan for their next meeting was to avoid pushing back and simply try to build a relationship with Ms. Peterson. Here is how the meeting went.

Dr. Blake sat down on the edge of Ms. Peterson's bed and said;

> *"I was wondering if we could talk for a few minutes about your care."*
>
> *"There is nothing to talk about. You people refuse to help me, so what is there to talk about?"*
>
> *"We aren't refusing to help you. We are refusing to help you die."*
>
> *"Same thing."*

Dr. Blake was frustrated again, but pressed on;

> *"Our job is not to kill people. Our job is to help people get better and relieve suffering."*
>
> *"Doesn't seem like you are doing your job too well here."*
>
> *"I <u>am</u> trying my best to help you. We are on your side."*

Ms. Peterson leaned back and closed her eyes. Dr. Blake's shoulders slumped and his head hung low as he left the room.

# Breaking the Cycle: From Helpless to Hopeful

Dr. Blake was once again caught in the Symptomatic Cycle. While his intention was to change the pattern of interaction with Ms. Blake, he got caught in the Symptomatic Cycle by responding directly to Ms. Peterson's provocative statement. This illustrates how difficult it can be to break the cycle. While he understood that a major part of the problem was Ms. Peterson's isolation, he needed more guidance. This is where the universal principles and the ARCH can help. The key principles to use include; focus on the relationship, highlight competencies, and be clear about your role, limits, and functions. The next day, he went to see her again.

## Focus on Relationships

Dr. Blake started his next meeting with Ms. Peterson differently.

> *"Ms. Peterson, I have been thinking a lot about our recent conversations. One of the things I've noticed about you is that people take a strong interest in you and your life. They get invested in you. (Highlighted the competency of being able to develop important relationships.) I'm very sorry that*

*your disease has come back and you see death as your only
option. I can see that your family cares deeply for you, and
you about them."*

Ms. Peterson does not respond, so Dr. Blake continues.

*"One of the things that troubles me, though, is that it appears that you are facing this challenge in your life alone."*
(Points out patient's isolation.)

*"So?"*

*"So, it must be hard to be thinking about your death and
have no one who you can talk to about it."* (Acceptance—
speaks in a non-judgmental way about her isolation.)

Ms. Peterson is once again silent. Her silence can be interpreted in many
ways. She may be angry, confused, or overwhelmed. Or she may not be experiencing any of those feelings. Dr. Blake waits a few moments and when
Ms. Peterson does not say anything, he continues to apply the universal principles and the ARCH in an effort to build his relationship with her.

*"Ms. Peterson, things must be very difficult for you right now
if you feel like death is your best option. I don't know what
you are feeling, but I trust it's pretty uncomfortable* (Acceptance). *I want you to know that even if I don't agree with
what you are asking for, I understand that you really do see
it as your best option* (Respect). *What I don't understand is
why you want us to help you die* (Curiosity)? *Quite frankly,
when you asked me to shoot you, it scared me* (Honesty)."

Dr. Blake has set a calm tone and has avoided getting caught in the Symptomatic Cycle again by accepting Ms. Peterson and by being curious rather
than controlling ("Ms. Peterson, you need to stop asking us to kill you. We
won't do it!"). Dr. Blake continued.

*"So, why do you want us to end your life?"* (Curious)

Ms. Peterson keeps her eyes closed and Dr. Blake waits for a few moments
and decides to leave. He has decided to leave her room on several prior occasions, but this time is different. In the past he left because either he was confused or angry. Today he is leaving because he feels like he has accomplished
what he can for now. He is neither frustrated nor angry.

*"Ms. Peterson, I am going to leave for now. I will be back tomorrow and I look forward to speaking with you again. If you
need me, just ask the nurse to page me."*

Dr. Blake left the room feeling surprisingly relaxed. His new framework of
trying to build a relationship and to be accepting of Ms. Peterson decreased

his frustration and directed his thinking toward how to connect with Ms. Peterson as opposed to how to get her to stop requesting help with her death. He ran into Ms. Peterson's nurse in the hall.

> *"How is the grim reaper doing today?" said the head nurse.*
>
> *"Medically, she is stable."*
>
> *"I know that. Did she ask you to bring in your hunting rifle?"*
>
> **Dr. Blake chuckles and says,** *"No, she didn't ask for that. I actually had a nice meeting with her."*
>
> *"Really?"*
>
> *"Yeah. She didn't say much, but I think I might be getting somewhere with her."*
>
> *"What's your secret?"*

Dr. Blake's secret was simply shifting his framework from control to collaboration. He was looking forward to his next meeting with Ms. Peterson. The next morning he entered her room and said,

> *"Good morning Ms. Peterson. How are you feeling today?"*

Ms. Peterson did not respond.
Dr. Blake sits down.

> *"I was thinking about our chat yesterday and it occurred to me that if you choose not to talk with me, I can't help you. I really do want to help you, but without your input, I can only guess about what you need."*

Ms. Peterson remains silent so Dr. Blake continues.

> *"I think it would help me take better care of you if I knew why you wanted me to kill you. If there is some..."*
>
> *"Because I can't breathe!"*
>
> *"Oh, um, really?"*
>
> *"Yes, really!"*
>
> *"Well, what do you mean?"*
>
> *"I mean I can't breathe! I have to think about breathing. Is that normal? It never was for me. It feels like I am suffocating."*
>
> *"I didn't realize that."*
>
> *"Well I sure did."*

*"Okay, there are lots of things we can do to help you breathe easier. Thank you for telling me. Is there anything else you want to tell me?"*

*"Look, I know I am going to die. But the one thing I can't stand is the thought of suffocating to death."*

*"So, that is why you asked me to kill you?"*

*"Yes. If you can't save my life, then the least you can do is not let me die in the worst way I can imagine."*

Ms. Peterson's respiratory distress frightened her so much that she was looking for ways to end her life. When this was explained to the staff, they knew what to do and quickly relieved Ms. Peterson's respiratory distress. Since the treatment of respiratory distress is relatively common and straightforward in an ICU, why then did the ICU staff miss something so basic? Part of the answer lies in Ms. Peterson's decision not to communicate with staff. Another part of the answer may lie in the power of Ms. Peterson's requests for death. The emotional upheaval generated by her requests was so distressing that it created a blind spot and distracted staff from their primary role of providing competent medical care.

The blind spot also created isolation among the staff. They often talked about how difficult Ms. Peterson was to care for, but they did not discuss their guilt over not being able to help her more. They could see she was suffering, but instead of using their competencies to try to resolve the impasse, they blamed her for the problem.

## Know Your Role, Limits, and Function

In Ms. Peterson's case, the staff felt powerless because, despite their best efforts, she continued to make clear, stark, and disturbing statements about her desire to die. Their feeling of powerlessness led to anger, and they began to feel incompetent, which furthered their isolation, not just from the patient, but also from each other. They expressed frustration and a global sense of powerlessness over "not knowing what to do." While well-intentioned, the staff were at a loss as to how they could effectively respond to Ms. Peterson's requests for death. They were adamant that they would not participate in assisted suicide, but felt shame over avoiding her.

A part of the solution involved helping the ICU staff clarify their role in Ms. Peterson's care. They knew that what they did best was to take care of critically ill patients. They helped patients to live, not die. Ms. Peterson, even though dying, was not technically critically ill. In short, she was in the wrong place. This realization lifted the staff's burden of guilt and feelings of having failed Ms. Peterson. Once the roles of the involved parties were clarified, the staff talked more openly about ways to help Ms. Peterson rather than trying to convince her to stop making provocative statements.

# Scenario Resolution

Ms. Peterson was transferred to the palliative care service of the hospital where staff were better trained to help her deal with her medical and psychological problems. By emphasizing the loving and supportive relationships in her family, her physician began a conversation about death that was tolerable for the family and allowed Ms. Peterson to serve as a guide. Ms. Peterson's two biggest fears were suffocating to death and dying alone. When her family understood how they could be helpful, they were able to access their preexisting competencies and they organized around-the-clock schedules to be with her. This also began a painful family discussion about where Ms. Peterson would like to die (at home versus in the hospital).

During Ms. Peterson's two-week hospitalization, her medical management was stabilized and she became increasingly articulate about her wishes for the end of her life. Her family, while grief stricken, could reframe their contributions. Instead of viewing themselves as powerless to alleviate her suffering, they recognized that they had an important role to play in her death. Family members remained close to Ms. Peterson despite the intense feelings that death can generate. Ms. Peterson was discharged home and received hospice care. Six weeks later she died, at home, surrounded by her family.

# Practice Points

1. **You always have something to offer.** Trust that your relationship with your patient can tolerate the anxiety or fear generated by death and that healing, unlike curing, continues until the end of life. Even in the face of feeling powerless to help your patient, you always have something to offer—yourself.

2. **Curiosity leads to discovery.** Remaining curious, as opposed to controlling, will lead to unforeseen discoveries.

3. **Look below the surface for the keys to competence.** When people behave in provocative and attention-seeking ways, it is usually an expression of a longing for a different type of connection. Underneath the behavior is fear, or hurt, or worry. Remaining patient and respectful can change the way people relate to you.

## Summary

The case of Ms. Peterson illustrates how interpersonal aspects of an ethical dilemma can be an integral part of resolving the conflict. The ethical dilemma of physician-assisted suicide was a mask for the struggle of a patient to get adequate palliative care and find a different way to relate to those she loved as she was dying. By using the symptomatic cycle to understand the problem, and then using the universal principles to guide the process, there was a shift toward building relationships and away from exhibiting controlling behavior. The medical staff could then concentrate on delivering medical care and being supportive, while family members became actively involved in caring for Ms. Peterson at the end of her life.

The process proposed here is not about trying to "get patients to change their minds." The systems approach is an attempt to frame the engagement of ethical dilemmas as a concurrent process of building collaborative relationships while exploring the salient moral issues. In this case, the request for assisted death was driven by the patient's fear and isolation. If Ms. Peterson actually wanted help in dying, the systems-based approach used here would have revealed that at some point. Although the initial response of the ICU staff was to frame the problem as an ethical dilemma, blind spots around the interpersonal aspects of the conflict led to an impasse. Using the symptomatic cycle to emphasize the competence of the patient, family, and medical staff, combined with efforts to build collaborative relationships to decrease everyone's isolation, helped move the dilemma to a more satisfactory conclusion.

# References

1. **Blackall GF, Green MJ, Simms S.** Application of systems principles to re-solve ethical dilemmas in medicine. J Clin Ethics. 2005;16:20-7.

2. **Bascom PB, Tolle SW.** Responding to requests for physician-assisted-suicide: "These are Uncharted Waters for Both of Us..." JAMA. 2002;288: 91-8.

3. **Lo B.** Resolving Ethical Dilemmas: A Guide for Clinicians, 3rd ed. Philadel-phia: Lippincott Williams & Wilkins; 2005.

4. **Micucci JA.** The Adolescent in Family Therapy: Breaking the Cycle of Con-flict and Control. New York: The Guilford Press; 1998.

# Chapter 10
# It's All In Your Head: Patients Seeking Medical Solutions to Non-Medical Problems

Daniel Sienna is a patient that some physicians would call one of the "worried well." At 71, he is married, has three grown children, and is retired from a career as a modestly successful corporate accountant. Overall, he is in good health. On the surface his life appears to be on cruise control. But inside, in his own words, he is "a total wreck."

Mr. Sienna has a pattern of developing a physical symptom (chest pain, abdominal pain, migraines, fatigue) that he believes to be a crisis. He then goes to his internist pleading for a medical intervention. Mr. Sienna's internist, Kelly Nash, has known him for two years and has struggled with how to help him. She believes that Mr. Sienna's main problem is that he has an anxiety disorder that is being manifested through physical symptoms.

**Key Terms**
- Blind spots lead to impasses
- Making mental health referrals

# "I Think I'm Having a Heart Attack"

Mr. Sienna called Dr. Nash's office on a recent Monday morning requesting an appointment. His main complaint was chest pain. The receptionist offered Mr. Sienna an appointment for that morning, but encouraged him to go to the emergency department if his symptoms got worse. Mr. Sienna insisted that he would "make it' until the appointment. Dr. Nash was concerned as she entered the room.

> "Hi Mr. Sienna, can you tell me what is happening?"
>
> "I have this pain right in the middle of my chest. It feels like a combination of burning and twisting."
>
> "When did the pain start?"
>
> "Friday night I was lying in bed and when I tried to turn over, I felt the first stab of pain."
>
> "Is it constant?"
>
> "No, it comes and goes."
>
> "Any shortness of breath or pain in your shoulder or down your arms?"
>
> "No, I can breathe fine and there's no pain down my arms. Actually, I did find myself a bit short of breath. I was breathing very fast."
>
> "Let me listen to your heart and lungs."
>
> "What do you think it is? I think I'm having a heart attack."

Dr. Nash starts to perform a physical exam and replies,

> "I don't know yet."

# No Stone Unturned

The initial physical exam was normal but Dr. Nash was concerned that there might be a cardiac problem so she ordered some tests and appropriate lab work. She tried to be calm and reassuring to Mr. Sienna.

> "Well Mr. Sienna, right now your physical exam is normal and your heart and lungs sound good. I do think, given that you are having chest pain, we should run a few more tests just to make sure we aren't missing anything. I think you should get an EKG, a chest x-ray, some blood work, and a stress test just to make sure we haven't left any stone unturned."

> "A stress test? Oh God, I knew it was bad. It's a heart attack isn't it?"
>
> "I didn't say that. I believe it is important to be thorough so that nothing is missed."
>
> "That's doctor-speak for 'you're a goner.' Oh man, I just knew it the second I felt the chest pain that it was big trouble. What will you have to do? Bypass surgery?"
>
> "Mr. Sienna, I think you might be jumping the gun a little bit here. No one is even thinking about surgery right now."
>
> "I am."

Mr. Sienna's anxiety was apparent but Dr. Nash felt compelled to investigate physical causes of his chest pain before she attributed it to anxiety. She felt he was overreacting to her assessment but also acknowledged that chest pain was frightening for most people. As she thought about possible causes of chest pain, she also considered how to encourage Mr. Sienna to get appropriate treatment for his anxiety.

Referring patients to mental health professionals was always a challenge for Dr. Nash. She worried about offending her patients but also carried the nagging concern that all physicians have about missing some physical cause for a patient's problem. With these thoughts running through her mind, she arranged for Mr. Sienna to obtain the appropriate tests and lab work. He returned one week later to get the test results.

> "Hi Mr. Sienna, I have good news for you. All of the test results were normal. Your heart is actually quite healthy."
>
> "Well that certainly is good news. That chest pain has actually gone away. But I started getting this terrible burning pain in my stomach over the weekend. It's right here (points to stomach). It feels like something is exploding in there. It comes out of nowhere and it is a searing pain. It takes my breath away. I was at the mall on Sunday and the pain was so bad I thought I was going to fall over."

Dr. Nash was surprised by Mr. Sienna's new complaint, but goes on to try to assess it.

> "Tell me a little bit more about the pain. Have you ever had it before?"
>
> "Never."
>
> "Well, we should look into this, but I don't think it's anything terrible."
>
> "How can you be sure? I had a friend a few years back who got colon cancer. The first symptom he had was the same

> type of pain. He only lasted one year once they figured out
> that it was cancer. It was terrible, in the end apparently it got
> into his liver and he turned all yellow. The pain was unbear-
> able for him."

> "I really don't think you have colon cancer. We can take a
> careful approach without jumping the gun and ordering in-
> vasive and expensive tests. I am optimistic that this is not
> something dreadful."

> "That is good to hear. Sometimes when I get these painful
> things I think I might be going crazy."

Performing a physical exam, Dr. Nash says,

> "You are not going crazy. This sounds like you might have an
> irritable bowel. I will prescribe a medicine that will help re-
> lieve any spasms in your intestines. I would like to see you
> back in three weeks for follow-up. If your pain gets worse, or
> if you have any other symptoms like blood in your stool,
> please call right away."

> "Thank you so much Dr. Nash. I can't tell you how much I ap-
> preciate you taking such good care of me."

## Physician-as-Expert?

Kelly Nash is slightly amused by the transient nature of Mr. Sienna's symptoms, yet also feels increasingly annoyed at his pattern of behavior. She feels
like her time is being wasted on someone with a psychiatric problem when
she has plenty of patients who are sick and need her medical expertise. This
leaves her feeling powerless because she does not know how to direct Mr. Sienna to the help he needs. While the model of the Physician-as-Expert is being enacted here (Figure 10-1), Dr. Nash feels more like a babysitter than an
expert. Up to now, she has been tolerant of Mr. Sienna's many complaints.
That is about to change.

## Let's Get a CAT Scan

When Dr. Nash entered the exam room for the three-week follow-up visit, Mr.
Sienna was sitting quietly in the corner.

> "The pain is no better Dr. Nash. I am really worried now. I
> know you said you didn't think this was anything bad, but
> how can we know for sure? I think we should get a CAT scan
> and find out just how big this tumor is."

**Physician-As-Expert Model**

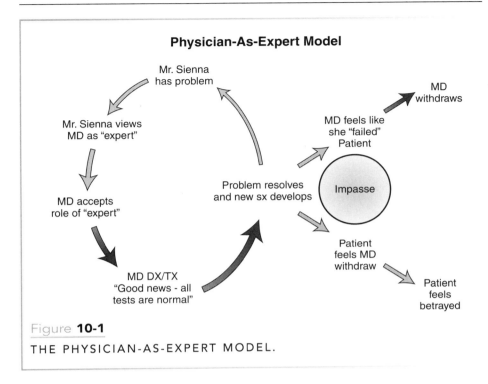

Figure **10-1**

THE PHYSICIAN-AS-EXPERT MODEL.

*"I don't think we need a CAT scan."*

*"MRI?"*

*"Mr. Sienna, let's not overreact to this pain. These tests are expensive and not medically indicated at this time. There are more conservative things we can do to try to help you."*

*Mr. Sienna has a sense of urgency in his voice when he says "The pain is keeping me awake at night. If you won't let me get the CAT scan, what are you going to do to help me? Do I need to find another physician?"*

*"No, you don't need to find another physician. I think we should stick with the anti-spasmodics and try some dietary changes to see if you get some relief. I would suggest increasing the fiber in your diet and reducing high-fat foods. Can you try that for two weeks and then come back and let me know how you are feeling?"*

Passively, he replies, *"I'll try it."*

## Blind Spots Lead to Impasses

Dr. Nash feels trapped. While she has diligently pursued medical explanations for Mr. Sienna's complaints, she also sees his anxiety as a significant contributing factor. So what is the trap? Is it Mr. Sienna's complaints? Or, is it her discomfort with directly addressing the emotional aspects of his medical problems?

Dr. Nash's uneasiness with addressing Mr. Sienna's psychological functioning has led her to focus on medical solutions to the exclusion of other types of interventions (for example, psychotherapy or support groups). The blind spot is that she avoids her own reluctance to refer for mental health care by relying on her medical expertise and externalizing responsibility for the problem to Mr. Sienna. She thinks, "if he would just go to see a psychologist instead of me, he would be fine. He is a healthy person!" While well-intended, Dr. Nash still misses the mark. Frustrated, she finally decides to address the issue with Mr. Sienna.

## "My Best Effort Backfired"

As Mr. Sienna was slowly getting ready to leave after his three-week follow-up appointment, Dr. Nash sensed his reluctance and felt that the conversation was not yet over. She decided to take a chance and bring up the issue of psychological factors in his medical complaints.

> "Mr. Sienna, there is one more thing I would like to speak with you about. I have noticed that you tend to be a worrier. Sometimes when we worry, our bodies react to the worry in uncomfortable ways. I think that your worries play a part in the physical symptoms you develop."

> "What do you mean?"

> "Your mind is messing with your body."

> "Are you saying I'm nuts? That this is all in my head?"

> "I am not saying you are nuts, but in a way, yes, I am saying that part of this is in your head. By that I mean that your anxiety ..."

> "Sure I have anxiety—wouldn't you? I'm 71 years old and I keep getting these medical problems. If these problems continue, who knows what could happen next? Then what is going to happen? I don't know what you are implying, but I am not making this up. I have serious pain in my stomach."

> "I know you have pain Mr. Sienna. What I am trying to say is that maybe seeing a psychiatrist could be helpful to you."

*"Psychiatrist? What does a psychiatrist know about stomach pain? I need a stomach doctor, not a head shrinker."*

Dr. Nash feels like her attempt to have Mr. Sienna see her perspective on the problem has backfired. Her first thought when Mr. Sienna gets defensive is "This is why I don't bring this psych stuff up." It also reminds her of when she developed migraine headaches while in medical school. She went to several different physicians and each one suggested that stress was the problem. She recalls how angry she got when the doctors tried to refer her to a psychiatrist. She felt humiliated and dismissed by the doctors. She never did go to a psychiatrist.

## Step 1: Seeing the Impasse

Dr. Nash is trapped. She believes that Mr. Sienna would benefit from mental health care, but is too uncomfortable to pursue the issue. She continues her conversation with him.

*"Mr. Sienna, I agree that there might be a role for a gastroenterologist in your care (reverting to the Physician-as-Expert Model). Actually, it has been on my mind lately. If you are not feeling better when you come back in two weeks, I think it would be appropriate to refer you to a gastroenterologist."*

*"Thank you. I just want to feel better."*

As Mr. Sienna left the room Dr. Nash thought to herself: "You are such a wimp." She felt like she backed down the minute the going got tough. Just like Mr. Sienna was trying to escape from his anxiety, she too was trying to avoid hers by taking the easy way out. Her discomfort drove her to compromise her professional beliefs. She did not believe that Mr. Sienna needed a GI consult. She did believe that he needed a psychiatric consult. As a result, she felt annoyed with Mr. Sienna and angry at herself. She was trapped in a cycle of frustration and conflict and has reached an impasse with Mr. Sienna. She was entrenched in the symptomatic cycle.

## Step 2: Understanding the Impasse

The Symptomatic Cycle (Figure 10-2) is the next step in helping Dr. Nash to understand why she is unable to steer Mr. Sienna toward mental health care.

As Mr. Sienna and Dr. Nash focus on seeking medical explanations and solutions to his complaints, their relationship begins to deteriorate and an impasse develops. The impasse is driven by Mr. Sienna's insistence on finding a medical explanation for his symptoms and Dr. Nash's reluctance to pursue psychiatric care for him. Mr. Sienna withdrew from the relationship because

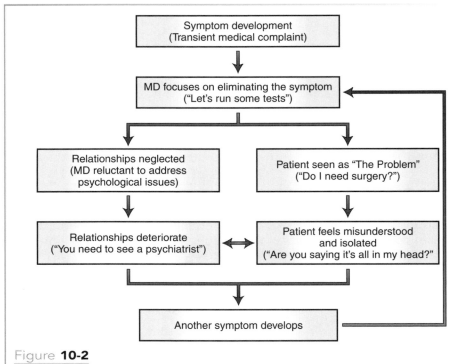

Figure **10-2**

SCHEMATIC OF HOW THE SYMPTOMATIC CYCLE WAS USED TO UNDERSTAND MR. SIENNA'S CASE (see text).

he was not open to Dr. Nash's ideas. Dr. Nash withdrew because she was hesitant to be open and honest with Mr. Sienna. While both parties have the same goal—for Mr. Sienna to feel better—the different beliefs create an opposing force that fuels the impasse (Box 10-1).

Box **10-1**

# Step 3: Responding to the Impasse

**1.** See your role in the impasse

**2.** Focus on relationships

**3.** Highlight competencies

**4.** Move from control to collaboration

# See Your Role in the Impasse

The first step in breaking the symptomatic cycle is for Dr. Nash to see her role in the impasse. She is reluctant to directly address the psychological aspects of Mr. Sienna's health problems because she does not feel competent in approaching her patients about the psychological factors in their health. One thing she can do to help herself is to connect with a trusted colleague who may assist her with this impasse.

# Focus on Relationships

As they become further entrenched in their positions, Mr. Sienna and Dr. Nash are feeling isolated and disconnected. Recommending that he see a psychiatrist is a sound thing to do. However, Dr. Nash's limited framework for explaining her position has worsened her relationship with Mr. Sienna. The first task for Dr. Nash is to decrease her own isolation with this problem. A good way to accomplish this is to talk with trusted colleagues. In this case, she decided to call one of her friends from medical school who is a psychiatrist.

> *"Hey, Paul, I need your help."*
>
> *"Hi, Kelly. So, you finally went off the deep end? I knew it was just a matter of time."*
>
> *"Glad to hear your sense of humor is intact and low-functioning. I have this case that is driving me crazy. It's a 71-year-old male who is in good health but he keeps returning with different medical complaints. When I work him up, everything is negative. He is highly anxious, and when I brought up seeing a psychiatrist, he didn't like it and then I backed down."*
>
> *"So, what's the problem from your standpoint?"*
>
> *"He keeps getting worked up for medical problems when the real issue is psychiatric. I simply don't know how to talk to him so that he doesn't get defensive and ask about needing more medical tests."*
>
> *"They never taught this stuff in medical school. I think it's good that you called me. My first question is, what is your framework for approaching him?"*
>
> *"What do you mean framework?"*
>
> *"What is your strategy for transitioning the conversation from exclusively medical to a broader framework that includes the mind and the body?"*
>
> *"I guess I don't really have one."*

Dr. Nash has accomplished several key tasks in this conversation. She has begun to decrease her isolation, and Paul has helped her to see one of the driving forces in the impasse; a lack of an effective collaborative framework to address the problem. The conversation continues with Paul trying to help Kelly access her own competencies.

> *"This is a common problem. You are a good internist and you have sophisticated strategies for treating all kinds of complex illnesses* (highlights competency), *but when it comes to matters of the mind, you have trouble applying what you already know. I think it might help you to think like an internist here, only apply it to the softer side of medicine."*

> *"What do you mean?"*

> *"Let's say he really did have a cardiac problem. How would you handle his care?"*

> *"Once I did a full diagnostic work-up, I would decide if I could handle his care or if he needed to see a cardiologist."*

> *"If he did need to see a cardiologist, how would you handle the referral?"*

> *"I would send him to someone I trust and then stay in touch with the cardiologist and my patient."*

> *"So you would continue to be his doctor?"*

> *"Of course I would! I don't dump my patients."*

> *"Does your patient know that?"*

Kelly pauses and feels a sudden sense of relief.

> *"In this case, probably not. When I mentioned seeing a psychiatrist, I rushed it because I was nervous and I was not clear that I would continue to be his physician."*

> *"When people get referred for mental health care, they often ask if they are crazy. What they really want to know is whether other people view them as being weak or in some way defective. The other thing they worry about is whether they are being abandoned. My guess is that the reason your patient went off was because he thought you were dumping him."*

> *"I see it now. Thanks."*

> *"No problem. I'm assuming your billing address hasn't changed?"*

> *"Wise guy."*

# Developing a Plan: From Control to Collaboration

Dr. Nash was feeling relieved because she began to understand her frustration and she felt an emerging sense of competence in her ability to work with Mr. Sienna. She also felt less alone with her problem. She knew she was not a doctor who dumped her patients and that was her starting point. With this new understanding, she eagerly approached her next meeting with Mr. Sienna.

> *"So, Mr. Sienna, how have you been feeling?"*
>
> *"Ok, except I have actually been having really bad headaches."*
>
> *"How is your abdominal pain?"*
>
> *"Pretty good actually. It has faded a bit. But these headaches are killing me. What do you think it could be? Not some kind of tumor, I hope?"*

Dr. Nash is surprised that she does not feel frustrated when Mr. Sienna presents yet another medical complaint.

> *"We can look into that, but first I wanted to talk with you about our last meeting. Do you remember when I suggested that you see a psychiatrist?"*
>
> *"Yeah."*
>
> *"Well, I have been concerned that in some way I offended you. If I did, please accept my apology. I feel like we need to back up a little bit here. You've had a number of different medical problems lately and we have not made much progress in figuring it all out. That said, I want to be clear that I want to be your doctor as long as you'll have me (focusing on the relationship). I think we both want you to live a healthy and productive life."*
>
> *"I do want you to be my doctor. But I agree we haven't made much progress."*
>
> *"I can tell that you are having a hard time with your health right now (Acceptance). It is also clear that you are working hard at getting well (Highlight competence). But, I have to admit that I am frustrated because I'm not sure if I am being helpful to you (Honesty)."*
>
> *"You help me a lot."*
>
> *"How (Clarifying roles)?"*

*"First, you agree to see me. I always feel like you listen to me. I do worry sometimes that I am frustrating you with all of my complaints."*

*"Sometimes I do feel frustrated (honesty), but it is not because of you. It is because I am trying to balance doing the right thing for you medically, with not overdoing it."*

*"I certainly don't want you to overdo it. But I still have these problems."*

Dr. Nash now has a plan that targets the deteriorating relationship with Mr. Sienna. Her goal in this meeting is not to get Mr. Sienna to agree to go to the psychiatrist. That would be an attempt to control him. But instead, she wants to decrease the isolation between them. Decreasing the isolation is an important part of disrupting the symptomatic cycle. She continues to try to focus on her relationship with Mr. Sienna by focusing on his strengths.

# Highlight Competencies

*"One of the things that I admire in you, Mr. Sienna, is your sense of responsibility* (Highlighting competence in an effort to shift the conversation away from deficits—"you're anxious"—to his strengths)."

*"Well, thank you. I do feel a strong sense of responsibility in my life."*

*"In many ways, that sense of responsibility carries over to your health. When you have a health concern, you do your best to get it taken care of* (Building the bridge between pre-existing competencies and current health problems)."

*"I never thought of it that way, but yes, I do want to get these problems taken care of."*

*"Good.* (Feels reluctant to take the next step of making a referral to a mental health provider—starts to revert to the Physician-as-Expert role.) *Can you describe your headaches for me?"*

*"Sure, they are usually on the right side, and the pain travels across the top part of my head and goes right into my eye. It throbs quite a bit."*

Dr. Nash performs an exam and does not have any significant findings.

*"Perhaps we should try some dietary changes like eliminating alcohol, caffeine, chocolate, and cheese for starters. The type of headache you are describing could be a migraine. It*

*may be linked to your diet or stress. I would like to see you
back in four weeks. If the headaches get worse, please come
in sooner."*

Using the universal principles has helped Dr. Nash to disrupt the Symptomatic Cycle. By moving the focus of the conversation away from medical
problems and symptoms, she has reminded Mr. Sienna about his pre-existing
competencies and how they apply to his current health concerns. While she
continues to feel reluctant to make a mental health referral, she has made
some progress disrupting the cycle and enhancing her sense of competence in
the interaction, thereby opening the door for a more collaborative relationship
with Mr. Sienna. When Dr. Nash feels engaged in a collaborative relationship,
she is free of the previous confinement of only talking about medical symptoms. In a collaborative relationship, she is able to freely talk about multiple
causes, and potential interventions, for Mr. Sienna's symptoms. Figure 10-3
shows how the Physician-as-Collaborator Model can be applied in Mr. Sienna's case.

In the Physician-as-Collaborator Model, Mr. Sienna and Dr. Nash work together to address the physical and the psychological aspects of his health. At

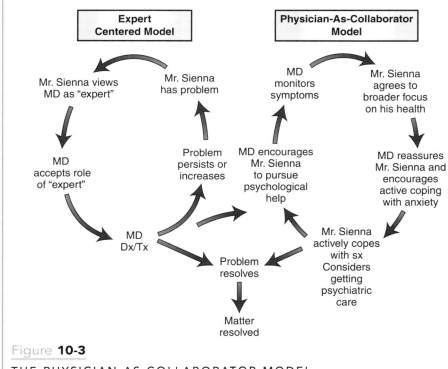

Figure **10-3**

THE PHYSICIAN-AS-COLLABORATOR MODEL.

this point they are not yet working in a collaborative manner. The barriers to a collaborative approach include Mr. Sienna's focus on his medical symptoms and Dr. Nash's reluctance to directly address the psychological aspects of his problems. Dr. Nash feels like she is making progress toward including Mr. Sienna's psychological functioning as part of the intervention, but still finds herself reluctant to refer Mr. Sienna for psychiatric services. She calls her friend Paul again to help unravel her reluctance.

# The Black Box

"Hi Paul, I have a few more questions about that case I mentioned last week. I did bring up the issue of anxiety as a possible factor in his illnesses in a way that did not result in him becoming defensive. But I still feel hesitant to actually make the referral to see a psychiatrist or a psychologist."

"Too bad, I could use the business—just kidding. What do you think is getting in the way of making the referral and feeling like it is the right thing for your patient?"

"I have been thinking about the cardiology example you used to illustrate how I would work in collaboration with another care provider to help my patient. As I thought more about this, it feels like when I do refer a patient to a shrink, they go into this black box and I never hear anything from the provider except maybe a brief note that the patient was seen and 'issues' are being addressed."

"Is that not enough?"

"No, because I feel out of the loop in my patient's care. I don't need to know every intimate detail of his personal life and his childhood..."

"We don't always talk about their childhood!"

"You know what I mean. I don't need to know everything, but it would help to feel like the psychiatrist and I are working together. Right now, when I refer to a mental health provider, I feel like I have lost control over my patient's care. My goal is not to turn over his care to another service. My goal is just like with a cardiologist—I make the referral and get input from the expert. The experts do their thing, but they stay in touch with me and they guide me on how I can improve my care of the patient."

"So, even though you make an appropriate referral, because you are not part of the process, it still feels a bit like a dump?"

*"Exactly."*

*"Sounds to me like you need to set some limits and estab-
lish expectations with your local psychiatrist."*

*"What do you mean?"*

*"Let me give you a few do's and don'ts."*

# Making Mental Health Referrals

The process of making mental health referrals has been covered extensively
by others (1), and Boxes 10-2 and 10-3 summarize some key things to do and
to avoid in this process.

---

Box **10-2**

## Do's for Making Mental Health Referrals

1. Be clear about what you see as the problem. "The patient has significant anxiety
   about his health. He also has multiple benign medical complaints." vs. "The patient has an anxiety disorder."
2. Be clear about your needs. "I need help on how to talk to my patient about the
   psychological aspects of his medical problems. I also need to be sure that my patient is receiving appropriate mental health care for his psychological difficulties."
3. Be clear about what you expect from the mental health provider (i.e., telephone
   contact, summary notes, periodic conversations).
4. Find several mental health providers who share your framework for helping people with medical and psychological problems.

---

Box **10-3**

## Don'ts For Mental Health Referrals

1. Don't put it off. The sooner you talk with your patient about this issue, the better
   off both of you will be.
2. Don't label your patient ("He's got a borderline personality disorder.") Labels are
   pejorative and do not contribute to a collaborative working process.
3. Don't refer to providers who work in a black box. You need helpful feedback.
4. Don't give up. If your patient initially refuses a mental health intervention, be patient and continue to build a collaborative relationship. You never know when he
   or she will feel ready for change.

# Mr. Sienna Returns

Before Mr. Sienna's next scheduled appointment, Dr. Nash started to think about how she was going to talk to him. In the four weeks since Mr. Sienna's last visit, she talked to several psychiatrists and psychologists recommended by Paul. She found one whom she felt would work collaboratively with her in Mr. Sienna's care. This psychologist also suggested some ways of talking to Mr. Sienna to facilitate the referral. Prior to entering the exam room she reminded herself of the principles that would guide her today (Box 10-4).

*"Hi Mr. Sienna, how are you today?"*

*"Pretty good. I changed my diet, but I still have headaches. I hope it's not a tumor."*

*"It is good to see that you are so motivated to get well by making the dietary changes (highlights competence). I admire how hard you work at that (Acceptance—she is not trying to change him—and Respect)."*

*"Thank you."*

*"You mentioned a tumor as a possible cause for your headaches. Have you thought about other possible causes (Curiosity—as opposed to "You don't have a tumor")?"*

*"My wife keeps saying it's because I worry so much. But I find it hard to believe that worrying could cause this much pain. I mean, there has to be something wrong up there."*

*"It is hard to imagine that worrying could create so much pain (Accepts his explanation as opposed to discounting it. Surprised that she feels so relaxed.). I mentioned to you several visits ago that something I struggle with is the balance between doing enough medical tests to make sure we aren't missing something versus doing too much and risking hurting you. I think these headaches are another example of this dilemma (Honesty). Based on my initial exam and your ex-*

---

Box **10-4**

## Guidelines for Talking with Mr. Sienna

1. Highlight his competencies
2. Use the ARCH- Acceptance, Respect, Curiosity, Honesty
3. Be clear about the physician's role, limits, and function

planation of the headaches, I don't think there is anything bad going on inside your head. That said, I understand that you are in pain. So the question is, what do we do next (Uses the term "we" to set the tone for a collaborative approach)?"

"I don't know. What do you think? You're the doctor."

"I am the doctor—that is true. And you are the patient, and the way I see it, we both need to have a say in how to keep you well. The last time you were in I said that I thought you were a very responsible person. I was wondering what you see as your responsibility in your health (Curiosity)?"

"I try to eat right and walk for exercise, but it is hard when my head hurts."

"Of course (Acceptance). Do you see it as part of your responsibility to explore different options to try to get yourself well (Curiosity)?"

"Yes. I would do anything to get rid of these headaches."

"Mr. Sienna, at this point, I see some limits to how I can help you. My bag of tricks can only take us so far. Quite frankly, I need some help here (Honesty). I think your body is pretty sensitive to many things. As hard as you try to be well (Highlights competency), you just seem to keep getting health problems. I will continue to try to find out what is causing your pain, but would you consider going to one of my colleagues—a psychologist—to see if he can help us (Curiosity and collaboration- "help us")?"

"Hmmm. I am not really fond of psychologists."

"Nobody is. All I am doing today is asking you to consider the option. If you decide that it is not an option for you, that is fine and we will continue to work together (Acceptance)."

"I will give it some thought."

"Thank you. Let's set up a follow-up appointment for four weeks."

# The Winds of Change

Dr. Nash felt energized after her last meeting with Mr. Sienna. Even though Mr. Sienna did not agree to see a psychologist, she felt like she was being a much better doctor. Because she had a plan and a sense of clarity in what she was doing (building a collaborative relationship, being curious rather than controlling), she felt a sense of accomplishment after the visit. Her competence in resolving the impasse was growing. She was so pleased that she decided to call Paul and share the good news.

*"Hey, Paul, I have some good news. I talked with that patient about possibly seeing a psychologist and it went pretty well. I was focused and relaxed and when I actually brought up him seeing a psychologist, he didn't get defensive."*

*"Good work. Maybe you missed your calling?"*

(Laughs). *"I don't think so. The strange part was that even though he didn't agree to go, I felt like I had accomplished something."*

*"Now you sound like a shrink—you talk to your patient and nothing happens and you take some perverse sense of delight in the conversation!"*

*"Is that how you guys do it? No wonder it's a black box."*

*"Actually, you did accomplish a lot. You have conquered one of your fears."*

*"So what do I do if he keeps refusing to see a psychologist or a psychiatrist?"*

*"What do you think?"*

*"You are such a shrink!"*

*"I try."*

*"I guess I just stay the course. If the goal is to develop a collaborative relationship with him, then being patient and accepting is the best way to get there."*

*"Exactly. At some point, something will change."*

*"When?"*

*"You are such an internist!"*

*"I try."*

## Scenario Resolution

Mr. Sienna eventually agreed to see a psychologist. The therapy helped decrease his anxiety. His medical complaints diminished but did not fully resolve. He continued to see Dr. Nash several times per year with different benign complaints. The conversation between Mr. Sienna and Dr. Nash had shifted from focusing exclusively on medical explanations for his complaints to a discussion of how his mind and body could work together to get him well. Dr. Nash truly enjoys working with Mr. Sienna. She also makes mental health referrals regularly. The mystery of the black box has been solved.

## Practice Points

1. **Face your fears.** Facing your fears will paradoxically lead you to uncover, and further develop, your competencies.

2. **Have a framework.** Talking with patients about topics that make us uncomfortable is never easy. Having a solid framework for the conversation (e.g., focus on building a relationship, allow patients to have their feelings, give a referral as part of working together) will help you to remain focused on the task at hand as opposed to being distracted by your feelings of anxiety or guilt.

3. **Stay connected.** Remind your patient that even though you are making a referral, you are still their doctor. They will appreciate your commitment, and being explicit will eliminate any question about your intentions.

## References

1. **McDaniel SH, Campbell TL, Hepworth J, Lorenz A.** Family-Oriented Primary Care, 2nd ed. New York: Springer; 2005.

# Afterword

Symptoms, systems, collaboration—by now you have the terminology mastered, and it is time to go out and use our models with your patients. Our teachers on these pages have been people whom we refer to as patients. Some of their lessons were easier to learn than others. Tom White required patience, while Julie Hennesy, the angry patient with back pain, demanded great self-restraint. Some of the cases had surprising twists and turns, such as Barbara Peterson, the young lady dying from metastatic sarcoma, or Mr. Thomas in the ICU. But in each case the treating physician was able to persist in the face of an impasse. However, persistence alone was not enough. They also had to be open and flexible enough to try a new approach to helping their patient. By using the Symptomatic Cycle, the Physician-as-Collaborator Model, and the universal principles, they found a way to resolve a troubling impasse.

Interviewing undergraduate students who are applying to medical school is an interesting experience. When asked why they want to pursue a career in medicine, at some point the answer includes "Because I want to help people." The answer is simple, often true, and, ultimately, gratifying. As years of clinical practice pass, though, the reasons you chose to practice medicine may become clouded by excessive demands, too many forms, and not enough time. We hope that by taking your valuable time to have read our book, you will have improved your skills in doing what we all try to do everyday: help people.

Since we started this book with the story of Bridget, it seems only fitting to end it with her. Bridget, the 12-year-old girl with leukemia, ended up being able to swallow pills. While she was trying all along to effectively learn how to swallow pills, the repeated frustration of failure drove a wedge between her family and the medical staff. It was through a combination of her practicing swallowing tic tacs and then gel caps that she developed the basic skills to take her medicines. But that was not enough. By helping the medical staff to become collaborative and not controlling, and by focusing on building a relationship with Bridget and her parents, their competencies flourished. Bridget's parents were able to lovingly set a limit, and Bridget's ability to focus and not give up eventually resolved the crisis. She became so good at swallowing pills that she later jokingly described herself as a professional pill taker. These same competencies, her focus and commitment, have led her to lead a successful life as a young adult. She agreed to let us use her story in the hope that it would instruct and inspire physicians to believe in their patients when they face an impasse. While her cancer is gone, the power of her struggle lives on. She was gracious enough to teach us. We hope that she has done the same for you.

# Index